WP HEALT

G000154576

VITαMINS

Know More About Vitamins, Minerals & Supplements

Tasha Jennings N.D.

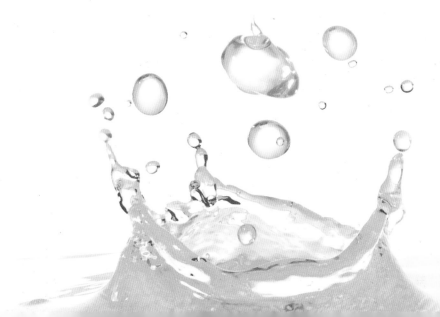

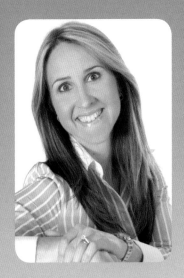

Tasha Jennings holds degrees in naturopathy, nutrition and herbal medicine and has over 10 years experience in the field. Tasha has extensive experience in clinical practice and is also an expert writer, trainer and presenter. Tasha is a regular keynote speaker at medical and health conferences and also runs trainings and seminars for medical and other health care professionals. She is an active and ongoing contributor to major media publications including newspapers, magazines, medical journals and websites. Continually inspired by innovative research in her field, Tasha progressed into product and program development and has been instrumental in the development of prominent vitamin and supplement ranges as well as a successful pharmaceutical health and weight loss program. Combining her clinical and business skills, Tasha recently established her own company Zycia, meaning 'life'. Zycia specialises in pre and postnatal nutrition to support life in its earliest stages and help provide optimal outcomes for mother and baby (www.zycia.com.au.) Tasha is now a new Mum herself and enjoys using her knowledge to inspire others to live healthier, happier lives.

Tasha Jennings
Bch H Sci Nat Med
Adv Dip Naturopathy
Dip Herb Med
Dip Nutrition

Published by
Wilkinson Publishing Pty Ltd
ACN 006 042 173
Level 4, 2 Collins Street, Melbourne, Vic 3000
Tel: 03 9654 5446 www.wilkinsonpublishing.com.au

National Library of Australia Cataloguing-in-Publication entry:

Author:	Jennings, Tasha.
Title:	Vitamins: Know More About Vitamins, Minerals & Supplements / Tasha Jennings
ISBN:	9781922178312 (paperback)
Subjects:	Vitamins. Dietary supplements. Vitamin therapy.
Dewey Number:	613.286

Photos and illustrations by agreement with international agencies, photographers and illustrators from iStockphoto.

Design: Jo Hunt
Printed in China

Contents

Introduction

I have been a Naturopath and Nutritionist for over 10 years and am passionate about spreading the message of good nutrition and the correct use of vitamins, minerals and supplements to help fuel your body.

Do you really need them?

Are you getting enough from your diet?

How do you know which ones to take?

Are you just paying for the latest 'fad'?

It used to be our local GP who recommended vitamin C for the common cold. These days, celebrities, not Health Care Professionals, often guide our supplement choices, with huge price tags attached!

Massive advertising campaigns and celebrity endorsements are taking over the vitamin market. But what are these supplements really doing for us?

This is vital information you don't get taught in school or by your Doctor, in fact, this is important information your Doctor might not know!

The nutritional material in *Vitamins: Know More About Vitamins, Minerals & Supplements* can not only add years to your life but also add life to your years (and to your wallet)!

This book will provide you with all the information you need to answer these important questions and navigate your way through the seemingly complex maze of nutritional supplements, past the advertising jargon and media hype, enabling you to make informed decisions about your health and your family's.

Tasha Jennings ND
Bch H Sci Natural Medicine • Adv Dip Naturopathy
Dip Herbal Medicine • Dip Nutrition

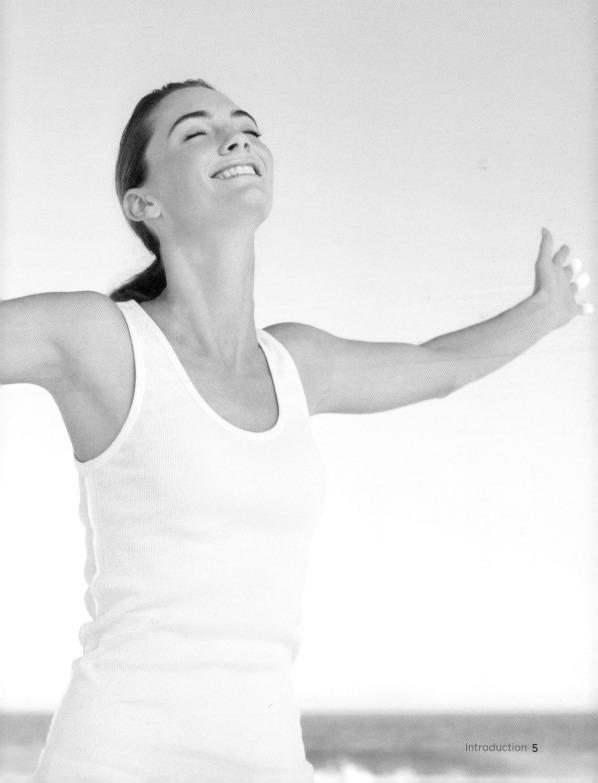

Vitamins and Minerals
The Lowdown

What are vitamins and minerals?

Vitamins and minerals are substances needed by the body for healthy growth and function. Some of these nutrients are key links in the chain of vital chemical pathways, activating nerve impulses, energy production and muscle contraction; others are essential building blocks for the development and maintenance of strong, healthy bodies.

These vitamins, minerals and other trace elements are known as micronutrients. The substances forming the larger bulk of our food, the protein, fats and carbohydrates, are known as macronutrients. Together the macro and micronutrients are the fuel which keeps our body running efficiently. Just like a car, the macronutrients can be seen as the petrol in our engine, and the micronutrients are the sparkplug, the battery and the oil. We need healthy balanced doses of all these essential ingredients to keep the motor running!

How much do we need?

Our Recommended Daily Intake (RDI) is a guide to the amount of each nutrient we should be consuming. However, in many cases we may actually require well above our recommended daily intake, with stress, lack of sleep and exertion increasing our demand for these nutrients.

Individual requirements also vary greatly due to factors including genetic makeup, inherited disease risk factors, metabolism, lifestyle, physical and emotional stress, pregnancy, smoking and age.

This means some people require larger/lesser doses of certain nutrients than others. So it's important to know how to identify deficiency signs and symptoms, to determine when you may need more or less of certain nutrients and what the ideal intake really is for you.

Too much of a good thing

Although it's essential to ensure an adequate intake of vital nutrients, it's just as important that they are not being consumed in excess. For some nutrients the upper safe limit (UL) is quite close to the Recommended Daily Intake (RDI) so excess intake should be closely monitored. Some nutrients are 'fat soluble', meaning they are metabolised and stored in our fat stores. These are not excreted by the body and can build up to toxic levels if consumed in excess. Other nutrients are water soluble and are rapidly metabolised and excreted from the body daily, therefore consumption well above the RDI is safe and actually recommended during times of stress or illness when our demand increases. Being aware of your upper safe limit of certain nutrients can be just as important as ensuring you have enough.

Where to get them from

A good healthy diet can provide a broad spectrum of vital nutrients and is the optimal source of essential vitamins and minerals. However it's important to be aware of which foods are the best sources of which nutrients. Unless you are consuming a wide variety of foods, even seemingly healthy diets can be lacking.

Dietary intake is also not the only factor involved in maintaining optimal nutrient status. These nutrients must not only reach the stomach but must also be absorbed into the bloodstream for them to be effective. Absorption of nutrients can be affected by a variety of factors such as illness, medications, metabolism, digestive health and interaction with other substances. For example, any conditions affecting the gut such as diarrhoea, irritable bowel syndrome, inflammatory bowel disease and celiac disease can hinder nutrient absorption. Common medications such as antacids, diuretics and the pill can also affect absorption. Even your daily coffee can hinder absorption of important nutrients while foods containing fibre can bind to some nutrients and affect uptake.

On the other hand, absorption of certain nutrients can be enhanced by the simultaneous consumption of other nutrients. Some vitamins and minerals are better absorbed via dietary sources, while others are actually best absorbed through supplements. By being informed and aware of these nutrient interactions and providing your body with the best sources to help ensure optimal absorption, you can quickly and easily maximise your nutrient status.

What about supplements?

Supplements will never and should never replace a balanced diet but appropriate nutritional supplementation can help bridge the gap between dietary consumption and the body's requirements. Taking a good multivitamin is like our insurance policy against deficiency and can help support optimal health, energy and vitality. Specific nutrients can also be used therapeutically to assist in the treatment of various diseases and conditions.

There is a vast array of nutritional supplements on the market, which supply a range of different forms of each nutrient. Some of these provide premium performance and lasting efficiency, while others offer little support and can even do more harm than good. It's important to know the difference. To ensure that you are getting lasting performance and the best value for money from your supplement, you need to know what to look for.

Terms Explained

RDI (Recommended Daily Intake)
The average daily dietary intake level that is sufficient to meet the nutrient requirements of nearly all (97-98%) healthy individuals in a particular life stage and gender group.

AI (Adequate Intake)
The average daily intake level, based on observed or experimentally-determined estimates of nutrient intake by a group (or groups) of apparently healthy people, that are assumed to be adequate. The AI is used when the RDI cannot be determined due to limited data.

UL (Upper Limit)
The UL is the highest average daily nutrient intake level likely to pose no adverse health effects to almost all individuals in the general population. As intake increases above the UL, the potential of adverse effects increases.

Antioxidant
Antioxidant refers to the ability of a nutrient to help protect our cells from oxidative damage caused by environmental exposure and the general effects of living and aging. While we're eating, digesting, exercising and even sleeping, metabolic functions occur which release free radicals into the system.

These free radicals are bullies! They love to attack and damage healthy cells. This leads to increased signs of cell damage, aging and can bring about changes in the cell which initiates cancer. Antioxidants are our cells' bodyguards! Once a free radical has been caught by an antioxidant, it can no longer cause harm and is simply excreted from the body. This is why antioxidants are commonly used in 'anti-aging' products and for cancer prevention.

All RDIs, AIs and ULs are based on Australian and New Zealand Guidelines.

Choosing a Multivitamin
YOUR ABC CHECKLIST

When choosing a supplement, it's important to remember that all multivitamins aren't created equal. Don't be fooled by fancy words or enticing imagery on the front of the label. The truth about your supplement is always contained in the nutritional panel on the back. To help you decipher the nutritional panel of your supplement, use our quick checklist below.

A. Does it contain all the vitamins and minerals I need?
Check the nutritional panel to ensure your supplement contains all the important nutrients your body needs for optimum health as outlined in this book.

B. Are the vitamins and minerals provided in adequate doses?
Some multivitamins may contain A-Z of all your nutrients but are they in a sufficient dose to be of benefit? Check the doses as outlined in this book to ensure your multivitamin contains enough of the important nutrients you need.

C. Are these nutrients supplied in well absorbed forms?
Vitamins and minerals can be provided in a variety of forms, some which are better absorbed than others. To make sure your supplement is well absorbed always check the nutritional panel to confirm that the nutrients are being supplied in well absorbed forms as outlined in this book.

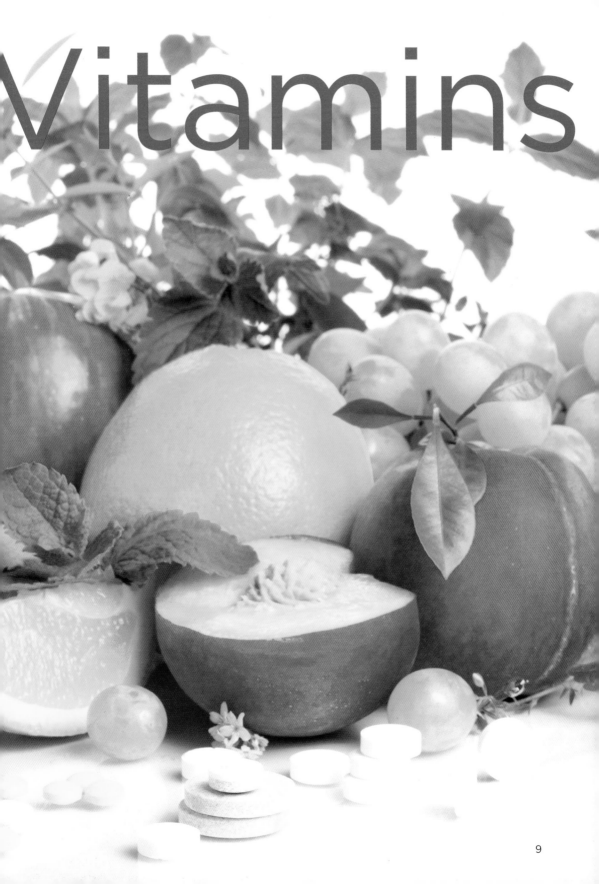

Vitamins

Vitamin A

The Snapshot

Vitamin A is an important antioxidant vital for healthy growth and repair of body tissues and especially important for eye health. Vitamin A is particularly involved in night vision, so the old wives' tale that carrots will help you see in the dark does hold some merit!

Available in the form of retinol or via beta-carotene, the pure retinol form is only available from animal sources and is the most active form. Carotenes, in particular beta-carotene, are a plant source of vitamin A. Beta-carotene is converted to vitamin A by the body when it's needed, helping avoid risk of toxicity.

Unless otherwise advised by a health care professional the safest way to consume vitamin A is through beta-carotene supplementation.

Other names

Retinol, beta-carotene, carotenoids.

What does it do?

Vitamin A is an antioxidant helping to protect cells from damage and reducing the effects of aging, and is vital for the growth, function and repair of bones, teeth, mucous membranes, skin and all skeletal and soft tissue.

Healthy functioning of the immune system relies on adequate supply of vitamin A to stimulate antibody response and white blood cell activity to help treat and prevent viral and bacterial infections.

The active form of vitamin A is known as retinol, due to its involvement in the production of retina pigments in the eye, which assist with vision. Vitamin A is also beneficial to help treat and prevent macular degeneration, particularly in combination with nutrients vitamin C, vitamin E and zinc.

With its role in growth and development, adequate vitamin A is essential for conception, pregnancy and breastfeeding. However excess vitamin A, particularly in supplemental form, can lead to birth defects, therefore intake should be contained within recommended doses during pregnancy and taken in the form of beta-carotene.

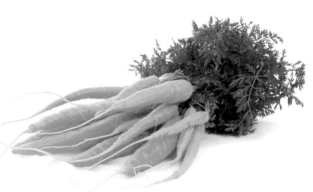

How do I know if I'm deficient?

Vitamin A deficiency is prevalent in developing countries however it is relatively rare in developed nations. Deficiency can be related to lack of intake of vitamin A containing foods, however it is more commonly related to lack of absorption. Being a fat soluble nutrient, absorption can be hindered by reduced ability to metabolise fats, as commonly occurs in alcoholics or those with liver disease, or a chronically low fat diet.

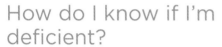

Signs and Symtoms

MILD DEFICIENCY
- Impaired vision, particularly night vision
- Impaired immune function
- Dry skin

SEVERE DEFICIENCY
- Blindness
- Hypokeratosis (hard bumps around hair follicles)

Is a supplement recommended for me?

Most good multivitamins will contain vitamin A, either in the form of retinol or beta-carotene. You can also find vitamin A or beta-carotene in good antioxidant combinations. Vitamin A is beneficial in conjunction with vitamin C, vitamin E and zinc for the treatment and prevention of macular degeneration. Unless deficiency has been established, single vitamin A supplements are rarely needed.

Which supplement should I choose?

Vitamin A comes in a number of forms; retinol, retinal, retinoic acid or retinyl ester. Unless otherwise advised by a health care professional the safest way to consume vitamin A via supplements is through beta-carotene supplementation, so your body only absorbs the amount of vitamin A it requires.

When should I take my supplement?

As a fat soluble nutrient, vitamin A is best taken with food.

What foods does it come in?

Liver	BETA-CAROTENE	Peas
Cheddar cheese	Pumpkin	Squash
Cod liver oil	Green leafy vegetables	Broccoli
Crab	Mango	Papaya
Carrots	Carrots	Nectarines
Egg yolk	Tomato	Spinach
Salmon liver oil	Apricots	Yellow vegetables
Milk	Peaches	Peppers
Butter	Collard greens	Cantaloupe
Halibut liver oil	Sweet potatoes	Watermelon

What happens if I take too much?

Unlike water soluble nutrients, fat soluble nutrients such as vitamin A are stored by the body and as such are more difficult to excrete, therefore it can accumulate. Excess consumption is not recommended and can lead to toxicity, causing symptoms such as nausea, irritability, loss of appetite, blurry vision, vomiting, abdominal pain, headaches, weakness, drowsiness, dry skin, liver damage, jaundice and hair loss. Vitamin A toxicity has been associated with increased fractures and osteoporosis due to depletion of the vital bone nutrients D and K.

Vitamin A intake should be particularly monitored in pregnancy as excess intake can harm a growing foetus. It is, however, essential to maintain adequate vitamin A levels for healthy growth and development of the foetus. Beta-carotene is the safest source of vitamin A to consume during pregnancy to maintain healthy levels without risk of toxicity.

Matching it up

TAKE VITAMIN A WITH

- Vitamin A can have a positive effect on the absorption of iron and zinc
- Zinc is also required to help transport vitamin A to where it's needed in the body
- Vitamin A works well in combination with vitamin C, vitamin E and zinc for the treatment and prevention of macular degeneration

DON'T TAKE VITAMIN A WITH

- Vitamin A can compete with vitamin D and K for absorption
- Avoid vitamin A in the form of retinol during pregnancy

How much should I have?

IU (International units)

IU is often used when referring to measurements of fat soluble nutrients vitamin A, vitamin D, vitamin K or vitamin E. One International Unit (IU) of vitamin A is equivalent to 0.3mcg.

INFANTS	AI	UL
0 - 6 months	250mcg/day (833IU)	600mcg/day (2000IU)
7 - 12 months	430mcg/day (1433IU)	600mcg/day (2000IU)
TODDLERS	**RDI**	**UL**
1 - 3 years	300mcg/day (1000IU)	600mcg/day (2000IU)
4 - 8 years	400mcg/day (1333IU)	900mcg/day (3000IU)
CHILDREN	**RDI**	**UL**
Boys 9 - 13 years	600mcg/day (2000IU)	1700mcg/day (5666IU)
Boys 14 - 18 years	900mcg/day (3000IU)	2800mcg/day (9333IU)
Girls 9 - 13 years	600mcg/day (2000IU)	1700mcg/day (5666IU)
Girls 14 - 18 years	700mcg/day (2333IU)	2800mcg/day (9333IU)
ADULTS	**RDI**	**UL**
Men 19 - 70 + years	900mcg/day (3000IU)	3000mcg/day (10,000IU)
Women 19 - 70 + years	700mcg/day (2333IU)	3000mcg/day (10,000IU)
PREGNANCY	**RDI**	**UL**
14 - 18 years	700mcg/day (2333IU)	2800mcg/day (9333IU)
19 + years	800mcg/day (2666IU)	3000mcg/day (10,000IU)
LACTATION	**RDI**	**UL**
14 - 18 years	1100mcg/day (3666IU)	2800mcg/day (9333IU)
19 + years	1100mcg/day (3666IU)	3000mcg/day (10,000IU)

THERAPEUTIC ADULT DOSE

The RDI of vitamin A is generally adequate to carry out most functions in the body, however to provide antioxidant activity in times of increased exposure to environmental pollutants or stress, doses at the UL between **3000 - 4000mcg** are recommended. Ideally this should be consumed in the form of beta-carotene. 6mg (6,000mcg) of beta-carotene is considered to be approximately equivalent to 1mg (1,000mcg) of vitamin A. This dose however is not recommended during pregnancy.

Vitamin B1

The Snapshot

Vitamin B1 is involved in many functions and processes in the body particularly the nervous system and the stress response as well as brain and memory function. It also forms part of our body's 'spark plug' and helps to convert our fuel (food) into active energy!

Thiamin is the only supplemental source of vitamin B1. Unless otherwise recommended by a health care professional, vitamin B1 is best taken in a supplement containing all the B complex vitamins.

Other names

Thiamin or thiamine

What does it do?

Vitamin B1 is involved in many body functions and processes, particularly in the nervous system. Adequate B1 is important to support nerve conduction and the stress response as well as brain function and memory.

Vitamin B1, as with other members of the B vitamin family, is important for carbohydrate metabolism and the conversion of carbohydrate into energy. Vitamin B1, in combination with all the B vitamins, is like the spark plug in a car. No matter how much fuel you put in, if the spark plug is not firing to get the fuel to where it needs to be, then you're not moving far! B vitamins help convert the fuel (food) we put into our body into active energy, which can then be used all over the body.

Vitamin B1 is also essential for the production of hydrochloric acid in the stomach, which is vital for healthy digestion as it kick-starts the fuel-to-energy conversion by breaking it down into smaller molecules, which are then metabolised and converted into active energy.

How do I know if I'm deficient?

Deficiency can be caused by a lack of vitamin B1 containing foods or diminished ability to absorb B1 from the diet. Very little vitamin B1 is actually stored in the body therefore consistent replenishment is essential as the body can become depleted within 14 days.

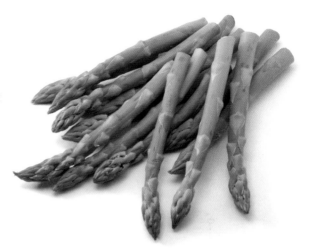

Signs and Symtoms

MILD DEFICIENCY

- Weight loss
- Fatigue
- Lack of concentration
- Mental confusion
- Irritability

SEVERE DEFICIENCY

- Severe eye fatigue
- Nervous system complications
- Muscle wasting
- Beriberi

The vitamin B1 deficiency disorder Beriberi affects the peripheral nervous system and/ or the cardiovascular system. If left untreated Beriberi can be fatal. This syndrome is mainly associated with severe malnutrition, gastrointestinal disorders, HIV/Aids and alcoholics where adequate B vitamin supplementation hasn't been administered.

What foods does it come in?

Pork	Sunflower seeds	Rye	Potato
Beef	Nuts	Wholegrain bread	Orange
Ham	Wheat bran	Wholegrains	Avocado
Lamb	Wheat germ	Peas	
Liver	Brewer's yeast	Corn	
Asparagus	Legumes	Broccoli	

How much should I have?

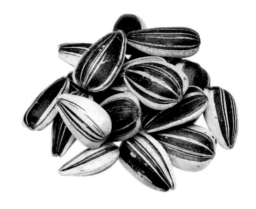

INFANTS	AI
0 - 6 months	0.2mg/day
7 - 12 months	0.3mg/day
TODDLERS	**RDI**
1 - 3 years	0.5mg/day
4 - 8 years	0.6mg/day
CHILDREN	**RDI**
Boys 9 - 13 years	0.9mg/day
Boys 14 - 18 years	1.2mg/day
Girls 9 - 13 years	0.9mg/day
Girls 14 - 18 years	1.1mg/day
ADULTS	**RDI**
Men 19 - 70 + years	1.2mg/day
Women 19 - 70 + years	1.1mg/day
PREGNANCY	**RDI**
14 - 18 years	1.4mg/day
LACTATION	**RDI**
14 + years	1.4mg/day

THERAPEUTIC ADULT DOSE

50 - 100mg/day is recommended to support the nervous system and energy production.
100mg - 300mg/day is used to treat deficiency and help repel mosquitoes!
Therapeutic doses of vitamin B1 should be taken in conjunction with a B complex supplement to ensure that all the B vitamins are maintained in balance.
There is no recommended upper limit (UL) for vitamin B1.

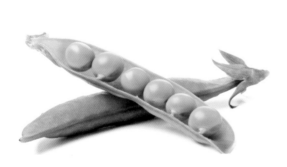

Is a supplement recommended for me?

Vitamin B1 supplements are often recommended for the elderly to help support memory and brain function. Supplementation is also recommended for recovering alcoholics. Vitamin B1 can be useful in combination with the other B complex vitamins for those lacking energy and/or under stress. B1 within a good B complex is also good for those taking the contraceptive pill.

Which supplement should I choose?

Thiamine (spelt thiamine or thiamin) is the only supplemental source of vitamin B1. For general health, stress and energy, vitamin B1 is best taken in a supplement containing all the B complex vitamins.

When should I take my supplement?

As with all B vitamins, vitamin B1 is best taken with food in the morning to avoid possible sleep disturbance at night.

What happens if I take too much?

Vitamin B1 has been shown to be safe even in high doses. No clear upper safe limit has been established however large doses may cause dermatitis, drowsiness or muscle relaxation in some people.

Matching it up

TAKE VITAMIN B1 WITH

- Diuretics can increase excretion of B1, increasing the body's demand
- The contraceptive pill can deplete the body of B1 so a vitamin B supplement is a good support for those on the pill
- Excess alcohol consumption depletes the body of vitamin B1
- B1 should be taken with a B complex supplement to ensure adequate balance

DON'T TAKE VITAMIN B1 WITH

- Antacids can reduce the body's ability to absorb B1
- Thiaminases, found in raw fish, shellfish and high sulfate foods can degrade B1, making it less available for absorption
- The flavonoids quercetin and rutin may hinder absorption of B1
- Single B1 supplements should not be taken long term unless combined with a B complex

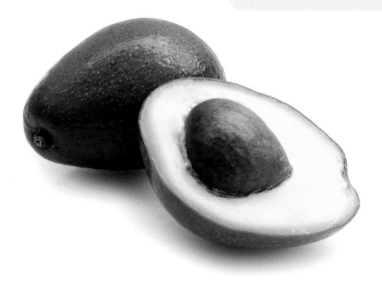

Vitamin B2

The Snapshot

As with all B vitamins, vitamin B2 is involved in the conversion of food to energy forming part of our body's 'spark plug'! It also plays a key role in the nervous system and stress response as well as aiding in hormone production and maintenance of healthy blood cells.

Vitamin B2 is known for its yellow-orange colour and because of this is often used as a natural food colouring (food additive number E101).

As a supplement, vitamin B2 should be taken in conjunction with a B complex containing all the B vitamins to ensure balance is maintained. But be warned, the metabolism of B2 will turn urine bright yellow! No need to panic, this discoloration is due to the natural metabolites being excreted and does not mean that B vitamins are being lost through urine.

Other names

Riboflavin

What does it do?

Vitamin B2 is essential for optimal body functioning at a cellular level. It plays a key role in energy metabolism by helping the body produce energy from the macronutrients protein, fat and carbohydrate.

Vitamin B2 supports healthy blood cells and is involved in iron metabolism, which further supports energy production. It's required for healthy development and function of the brain and nervous system and is involved in adrenal gland function and stress response.

Vitamin B2 is also involved in hormone production and regulation via its adrenal gland activity.

How do I know if I'm deficient?

Mild deficiency is relatively common if dietary sources are lacking as B2 is quickly lost from the body and thus requires constant replenishment. Deficiency of B2 is often accompanied by deficiencies of other B vitamins and can be quickly and easily corrected with supplementation or a few extra serves of your favourite vitamin B2 containing foods!

What foods does it come in?

Milk	Beef	Spinach	Whole grains
Yoghurt	Tuna	Eggs	Currants
Cheese	Organ meats	Wholegrain bread	Sprouts
Pork	Broccoli	Wholegrain cereal	Yeast

Is a supplement recommended for me?

Supplementation is recommended for those with cracks in the corners of the mouth. It is also recommended in combination with the other B complex vitamins for those lacking energy and under stress.

Which supplement should I choose?

Riboflavin is the only supplemental source of vitamin B2. Unless otherwise recommended by a health care professional, vitamin B2 is best taken in a supplement containing all the B complex vitamins.

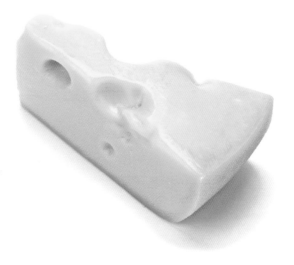

How much should I have?

INFANTS	AI
0 – 6 months	0.3mg/day
7 – 12 months	0.4mg/day
TODDLERS	RDI
1 – 3 years	0.5mg/day
4 – 8 years	0.6mg/day
CHILDREN	RDI
Boys 9 – 13 years	0.9mg/day
Boys 14 – 18 years	1.3mg/day
Girls 9 – 13 years	0.9mg/day
Girls 14 – 18 years	1.1mg/day
ADULTS	RDI
Men 19 – 70 years	1.3mg/day
Men 70 + years	1.6mg/day
Women 19 – 70 years	1.1mg/day
Women 70 + years	1.3mg/day
PREGNANCY	RDI
14 + years	1.4mg/day
LACTATION	RDI
14 + years	1.6mg/day

THERAPEUTIC ADULT DOSE

10 – 30mg/day is generally recommended and should be taken in conjunction with a B complex supplement.
There is no recommended upper limit (UL) for vitamin B2.

When should I take my supplement?

All B vitamins are best taken with food in the morning unless you're looking for an energy boost at night!

What happens if I take too much?

Risk of vitamin B2 toxicity is very low as the body will generally only absorb the amount it requires, meaning high dose supplements actually aren't absorbed above the amount that the body needs.

Matching it up

TAKE VITAMIN B2 WITH
• B complex

DON'T TAKE VITAMIN B2 WITH
• Single B2 supplements should not be taken long term unless combined with a B complex

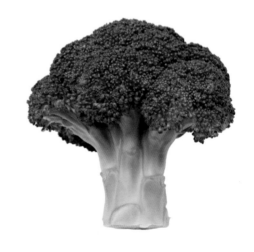

Vitamin B3

The Snapshot

As a member of the B vitamin family, B3 is a part of the body's 'spark plug', playing a key role in the conversion of food to energy as well as supporting the nervous system. B3 is involved in hormone production including the sex hormones, thyroid hormones and insulin.

Other names

Niacin, nicotinic acid, nicotinamide

These terms are often used interchangeably as they all function as vitamin B3, however they are metabolised in slightly different ways. Niacin takes an extra step in the conversion chain being converted to nicotinamide in the body before it's used.

What does it do?

As with all B vitamins, vitamin B3 is involved in healthy digestion and the conversion of food to energy. It plays a role in the healthy functioning of the nervous system and stress response.

B3 is involved in the production of hormones including sex hormones, the thyroid hormone thyroxin and insulin. Not only does vitamin B3 assist in the synthesis of insulin, it also forms part of the glucose tolerance factor. Glucose tolerance factor works with insulin to help transport glucose to cells efficiently, helping to regulate blood sugar and reduce sugar cravings!

Niacin supplementation can assist in the reduction of cholesterol, in particular the bad LDL cholesterol, as well as helping reduce atherosclerosis (hardening of the arteries).

How do I know if I'm deficient?

Deficiency is uncommon in developed countries tending to be more associated with those experiencing chronic malnutrition or in alcoholics, as alcohol can deplete B vitamins.

Symptoms of pellagra include digestive upset; diarrhoea, dermatitis, thickening of the skin and 'necklace' like lesions around the neck, painful inflamed mouth and tongue as well as mental disturbance including dementia and delirium. If left untreated, pellagra can be fatal.

Signs and Symtoms

MILD DEFICIENCY

- Decreased metabolism
- Decreased tolerance to cold
- Anxiety/depression
- Listlessness/poor concentration

SEVERE DEFICIENCY

- Pellagra

What foods does it come in?

Tuna	Beef	Legumes	Brown rice
Turkey	Pork	Peanuts	Bread
Chicken	Salmon	Sunflower seeds	Milk
Fish	Sardines	Asparagus	Yoghurt
Veal	Scallops	Wheat germ	Cottage cheese
			Yeast

Is a supplement recommended for me?

Therapeutic doses of niacin can be beneficial for those with high cholesterol. Vitamin B3 in combination with the other B complex vitamins can be also be useful for those with low energy and/or under high stress.

Which supplement should I choose?

If using to help reduce cholesterol, you should look for a supplement containing 1000mg - 2000mg of vitamin B3 in the form of niacin, taken 3 times per day. In a B complex to help support energy, nicotinamide is a better option for easier absorption.

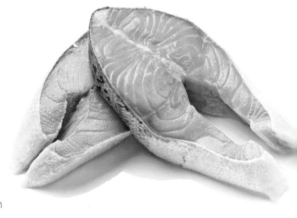

How much should I have?

INFANTS	AI
0 – 6 months	2mg/day
7 – 12 months	4mg/day
TODDLERS	RDI
1 – 3 years	6mg/day
4 – 8 years	8mg/day
CHILDREN	RDI
Boys 9 – 13 years	12mg/day
Boys 14 – 18 years	16mg/day
Girls 9 – 13 years	12mg/day
Girls 14 – 18 years	14mg/day
ADULTS	RDI
Men 19 – 70+ years	16mg/day
Women 19 – 70+ years	14mg/day
PREGNANCY	RDI
14 + years	18mg/day
LACTATION	RDI
14 + years	17mg/day

THERAPEUTIC ADULT DOSE

50 – 150mg/day is recommended to support energy and hormone production.

100 - 200mg is recommended to support insulin function and blood sugar control.

3000-6000mg/day of niacin is recommended to help lower cholesterol. This dose should be divided into 1,000 – 2,000mg 3 x per day. Therapeutic dosing of niacin can cause flushing in some people.

There is no recommended upper limit (UL) for vitamin B3.

When should I take my supplement?

As with all B vitamins, vitamin B3 should be taken in conjunction with the whole B group family and should be taken with food in the morning. If using single high dose supplements for cholesterol reduction, an additional B complex supplement should be taken alongside it. Taking niacin supplements with food can help reduce the flushing side effects.

What happens if I take too much?

Treatment doses of niacin of 1000mg or more will generally cause some degree of flushing, which will usually subside once the dose has been administered consistently for a few weeks. Excess niacin can also be associated with headaches and digestive upset. Niacin can assist glucose tolerance however excess doses can actually upset blood sugar balance in some people, which is particularly important for diabetics. Taking vitamin B3 in the form of nicotinamide will not elicit any of these toxicity effects.

Matching it up

TAKE VITAMIN B3 WITH
- B complex

DON'T TAKE VITAMIN B3 WITH
- High doses of B3 in the form of niacin should be avoided by diabetics due to possible impairment of blood glucose levels
- Single B3 supplements should not be taken long term unless combined with a B complex

Vitamin B5

The Snapshot

As with the other members of the B vitamin family, vitamin B5 forms part of our metabolic 'spark plug' and is involved in the conversion of food to energy as well as supporting the nervous system and stress response. B5 also helps improve hair health and growth.

Vitamin B5 is best taken in combination with the other B vitamins and single supplementation is rarely required.

Other names

Pantothenic acid, pantothenate

What does it do?

Vitamin B5 is involved in the metabolism of carbohydrate, fat and protein and its conversion to energy. It is essential for the healthy functioning of the nervous system and is involved in the production of adrenal hormones, which assist in the body's stress response.

Vitamin B5 can penetrate the cortex of the hair and may help improve strength and growth.

How do I know if I'm deficient?

Vitamin B5 deficiency is exceptionally rare, however when registered is quickly and easily reversed via supplementation or a good helping of vitamin B5 containing foods.

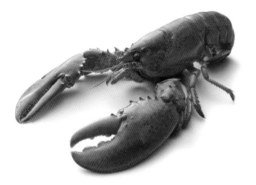

Signs and Symtoms

MILD DEFICIENCY

- Burning feet
- Irritability
- Restlessness/sleep disturbance
- Headaches
- Fatigue
- Nausea/vomiting
- Cramping
- Numbness
- Hypoglycaemia

SEVERE DEFICIENCY

- No severe deficiency symptoms noted

What foods does it come in?

Beans	Liver	Yeast	Wholegrain cereal
Lentils	Lobster	Milk	Green leafy vegetables
Kidneys	Avocado	Blue cheese	
Heart	Mushrooms	Orange	
Brains	Peas	Wholegrain bread	

Is a supplement recommended for me?

Vitamin B5 as a single supplement is rarely required. It is generally recommended in combination with the other B complex vitamins for those suffering fatigue or stress.

Which supplement should I choose?

Calcium pantothenate and pantothenic acid are the most common supplemental sources of vitamin B5. Both are derived from the same source and perform the same functions. There is little evidence to suggest whether one is better than the other.

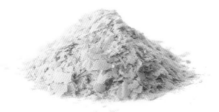

How much should I have?

INFANTS	AI
0 – 6 months	1.7mg/day
7 – 12 months	2.2mg/day
TODDLERS	AI
1 – 3 years	3.5mg/day
4 – 8 years	4mg/day
CHILDREN	AI
Boys 9 – 13 years	5mg/day
Boys 14 – 18 years	6mg/day
Girls 9 – 13 years	4mg/day
Girls 14 – 18 years	4mg/day
ADULTS	AI
Men 19 – 70 years	6mg/day
Women 19 - 70 years	4mg/day
PREGNANCY	AI
14 + years	5mg/day
LACTATION	AI
14 + years	6mg/day

THERAPEUTIC ADULT DOSE

25 - 100mg is a good dose to support general health and energy.

250mg – 1,000mg can be used therapeutically but this is best divided into smaller doses over the day for best absorption.

There is no recommended daily intake (RDI) or upper limit (UL) for vitamin B5. Recommendations are based on the adequate intake (AI).

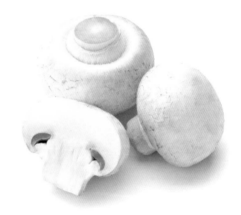

When should I take my supplement?

Vitamin B5 is best taken with food in the morning to avoid sleep disturbance at night.

What happens if I take too much?

There is virtually no toxicity with vitamin B5 and no upper tolerable limit has been established. The only side effect of massive excess consumption has shown to be mild intestinal discomfort and the effects of depletion of other B vitamins due to the excess single B supplement causing an imbalance in the levels of the other members of the B complex family.

Matching it up

TAKE VITAMIN B5 WITH
- B complex

DON'T TAKE VITAMIN B5 WITH
- Single B5 supplements are rarely required and should not be taken long term unless combined with a B complex

Vitamin B6

The Snapshot

Vitamin B6 plays a role in almost all processes in the body as it supports metabolic pathways at a cellular level. It plays a role in the health of the nervous system and stress response and is also essential for cardiovascular health, blood pressure regulation, a healthy immune system and hormone regulation.

Supplements can be beneficial in the treatment of PMS/PMT, to support cardiovascular health as well as for those lacking energy or under stress. As with all B vitamins, single supplementation should be taken in conjunction with a B complex.

Other names

Pyridoxine, piridoxal, pridoxamine

All three forms are broken down to the active form pyridoxal 5-phosphate and carry out the same functions in the body. Supplements are most commonly found in the form of pyridoxine hydrochloride.

What does it do?

As with the other B vitamins B6 is a vital part of the body's metabolic 'spark plug', involved in the release of energy from food. Vitamin B6 is particularly essential for protein metabolism.

Vitamin B6 is essential for hormone production and regulation and can be beneficial for the treatment of PMS and PMT, particularly for those taking the pill, which can deplete your body of vitamin B6. It can also help alleviate the symptoms of morning sickness in pregnancy.

Healthy functioning of the nervous system relies on vitamin B6 for the production of serotonin, dopamine and noradrenaline, all of which play a major role in mood regulation, assisting in the treatment of some forms of depression and helping to regulate mood swings associated with PMS or PMT.

Vitamin B6 is involved in the regulation of blood pressure and general healthy functioning of the heart. It can help prevent heart disease by assisting in the prevention of plaque build up in the arteries, helping to regulate blood pressure and cholesterol and prevent platelet aggregation. It also works in conjunction with B12 and folate to help reduce homocysteine levels, which can damage the artery walls and also increase the risk of blood clots. Our red blood cells rely on vitamin B6 for the synthesis of haemoglobin, which helps blood cells carry oxygen around the body.

Vitamin B6 is involved in the production of white blood cells which are vital to the healthy functioning of the immune system. Just like vitamin A, B6 helps prime the immune system for pending attacks!

Vitamin B6 also plays a role in the maintenance of healthy hair, nails and skin and can assist in the treatment of hormonal acne.

How do I know if I'm deficient?

Vitamin B6 is readily available in the diet and therefore clinical deficiency is rare in developed countries. However, those taking the contraceptive pill and those consuming a high protein or high sugar diet can be at greater risk of mild to moderate deficiency as demand for and excretion of B6 is higher in these circumstances.

Demand for and importance of adequate levels of B6 increases in pregnancy. Inadequate levels during pregnancy can cause fluid retention, nausea and vomiting and can increase the likelihood of developing blood sugar problems. Inadequate levels later in pregnancy have been associated with birthing difficulties.

Signs and Symtoms

MILD DEFICIENCY
- Dermatitis
- Depression
- Confusion
- Fluid retention (especially in pregnancy)
- Nausea/vomiting (especially in pregnancy)
- Birthing difficulties in pregnancy

SEVERE DEFICIENCY
- Mycrocytic anaemia
- Convulsions

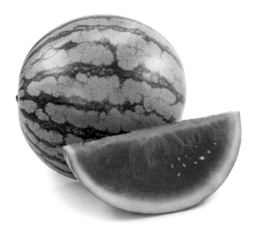

What foods does it come in?

Liver	Veal	Peanuts	Potato
Fish	Pork	Walnuts	Sweet potato
Salmon	Beef	Sunflower seeds	Carrots
Tuna	Eggs	Avocado	Peas
Mackerel	Lentils	Watermelon	Wholegrain bread
Chicken	Split peas	Bananas	Wholegrain cereal
Ham	Kidney beans	Brussels sprouts	

Is a supplement recommended for me?

Vitamin B6 supplementation is often recommended for those with hormonal imbalance or suffering PMS/PMT. It can be useful to improve hormonal acne and to support cardiovascular health. It is also beneficial, along with the other members of the B vitamin family, to help boost energy and in times of stress.

Which supplement should I choose?

Vitamin B6 supplements are found in the form of pyridoxine hydrochloride.

When should I take my supplement?

As with all B vitamins, vitamin B6 is best taken with food. As they are part of the metabolic 'spark plug' to help support energy production and keep the body firing, all B vitamins are also best taken in the morning, unless you're looking for some extra night time energy!

What happens if I take too much?

Excess consumption of vitamin B6 can affect the nervous system, resulting in neuropathy. This is generally only seen when doses of 2,000 – 5,000mg are consumed and can usually be reversed when supplementation is ceased. Therapeutic supplemental doses over 100mg per day should not be taken long term unless under the direction of a health care professional.

Matching it up

TAKE VITAMIN B6 WITH
• B complex

DON'T TAKE VITAMIN B6 WITH
• Single B6 supplements should not be taken long term unless combined with a B complex

How much should I have?

INFANTS	AI	UL
0 - 6 months	0.1mg/day	Not possible to establish
7 - 12 months	0.3mg/day	Not possible to establish
TODDLERS	RDI	UL
1 - 3 years	0.5mg/day	15mg
4 - 8 years	0.6mg/day	20mg
CHILDREN	RDI	UL
Boys 9 - 13 years	1mg/day	30mg/day
Boys 14 - 18 years	1.3mg/day	40mg/day
Girls 9 - 13 years	1mg/day	30mg/day
Girls 14 - 18 years	1.2mg/day	40mg/day
ADULTS	RDI	UL
Men 19 - 50 years	1.3mg/day	50mg/day
Men 50 + years	1.7mg/day	50mg/day
Women 19 - 50 years	1.3mg/day	50mg/day
Women 50 + years	1.5mg/day	50mg/day
PREGNANCY	RDI	UL
14 - 18 years	1.9mg/day	40mg/day
18 - 50 years	1.9mg/day	50mg/day
LACTATION	RDI	UL
14 - 18 years	2mg/day	40mg/day
18 - 50 years	2mg/day	50mg/day

THERAPEUTIC ADULT DOSE

30mg has been found to be a beneficial dose for assisting symptoms of morning sickness.

5 - 50mg is a good dose for general health and energy support.

50 - 100mg is recommended for the treatment of PMS and PMT and doses of **up to 250mg** have been used to treat hormonal imbalances. This dose is also beneficial for cardiovascular support. Doses above 50mg per day should not be taken long term and doses above 100mg per day should only be taken on the advice of a health care practitioner.

Biotin

The Snapshot

Biotin is like the 'black sheep' of the B vitamin family, so removed that it rarely goes by its lesser known name, vitamin B7. However, it still acts like a B vitamin by forming a part of our metabolic 'spark plug'. It also plays a role in the regulation of blood sugar and helps support the health of hair, skin and nails.

Biotin supplements can be beneficial in combination with the other B vitamins during times of stress or fatigue. Biotin is recommended during pregnancy and is also beneficial for the treatment of cradle cap in infants when taken by breastfeeding mothers. Supplementation can also be beneficial in the treatment of dermatitis, dry skin or brittle nails. Even as an alienated member of the family, biotin supplements are still best taken in conjunction with the other B group family members.

Other names

Vitamin B7, vitamin H

What does it do?

Biotin acts as a coenzyme in the metabolism of fatty acids, protein and amino acids and is involved in the production of energy. It plays a role in gluconeogenesis, which is a process by which the liver releases glucose back into the blood stream when stores are low, helping to maintain blood sugar balance and provide energy.

Biotin assists in the maintenance of healthy skin and nails by helping renew and replenish the outer fatty layer of our cells to prevent dryness. It can also encourage hair growth and help prevent hair loss.

Studies indicate that mild biotin deficiency is quite common amongst pregnant women, most likely due to the increased nutritional demand. Animal studies have linked biotin deficiency with birth defects and although this is not confirmed in humans, adequate consumption during this time is highly recommended.

How do I know if I'm deficient?

Deficiency of biotin is fairly rare. It is thought to be produced by the body in sufficient amounts to meet metabolic requirements if dietary sources are low; however it is unclear how well this source is utilised by the body. With many people suffering disruptions in healthy gut bacteria through stress, antibiotic use and exposure to bacterial pathogens this natural supply may be disrupted.

Deficiency has shown to be more prevalent in pregnancy, which can lead to an increased risk of birth defects. Those consuming large amounts of egg white in the diet can also be at greater risk of deficiency as egg whites can deplete biotin levels.

Signs and Symtoms

MILD DEFICIENCY

- Dry skin
- Dermatitis
- Hair loss
- Cradle cap in infants
- Muscle cramps after exertion

SEVERE DEFICIENCY

- Decreased muscle coordination and tone
- Seizures
- Possible birth defects

What foods does it come in?

Liver	Carrots	Cucumber	Raspberries
Egg yolk	Almonds	Cauliflower	Walnuts
Tomato	Onions	Milk	Oats
Romaine lettuce	Cabbage	Strawberries	Halibut

Is a supplement recommended for me?

Biotin supplementation can be beneficial during pregnancy. Those suffering dermatitis and dry skin can benefit from supplementation and supplements can also be given to the breastfeeding mother to assist in the treatment of cradle cap in infants. Biotin supplements can be useful for people experiencing hair loss, but be careful when paying top price for expensive shampoos containing biotin as there is little evidence to suggest that it's absorbed well through the skin, if at all!

Biotin can be useful in combination with the other B complex vitamins during times of stress or fatigue and in combination with magnesium to help treat post exertion muscular cramps and spasms.

Which supplement should I choose?

The only known biologically active form of biotin is D-biotin which is found in most dietary supplements. Most multivitamin and B complex vitamin supplements will contain biotin and it can also be found in some hair, skin and nail vitamin formulas. Biotin can be

How much should I have?

INFANTS	AI
0 - 6 months	5mcg/day
7 - 12 months	6mcg/day

TODDLERS	AI
1 - 3 years	8mcg/day
4 - 8 years	12mcg/day

CHILDREN	AI
Boys 9 - 13 years	20mcg/day
Boys 14 - 18 years	30mcg/day
Girls 9 - 13 years	20mcg/day
Girls 14 - 18 years	25mcg/day

ADULTS	AI
Men 19 - 70 + years	30mcg/day
Women 19 - 70 + years	25mcg/day

PREGNANCY	AI
14 + years	30mcg/day

LACTATION	AI
14 + years	35mcg/day

THERAPEUTIC ADULT DOSE

3,000 - 6,000mcg/day is generally recommended for the treatment of brittle nails, skin conditions and energy and nervous system support.

300mcg/day is recommended in pregnancy to prevent and treat deficiency.

6,000mcg/day can be given to the lactating mother to treat cradle cap.

7,000mcg - 15,000mcg/day is recommended if biotin is being used to assist the regulation of blood sugar.

There is no recommended daily intake (RDI) or upper limit (UL) for biotin. Recommendations are based on the adequate intake (AI).

What happens if I take too much?

Biotin is a very safe nutrient. There are no reports of biotin toxicity and no upper safe limit has been set.

taken as a single supplement, however these are rarely recommended as biotin works better in conjunction with other supportive nutrients.

When should I take my supplement?

As with the other members of the B vitamin family, biotin is best taken and absorbed with food. Due to its involvement in energy production, it is also recommended to take in the morning to avoid any sleep disturbance at night.

Matching it up

TAKE BIOTIN WITH
- Magnesium to assist with muscle cramps
- B complex
- Vitamin B5. These nutrients work together in many metabolic functions

DON'T TAKE BIOTIN WITH
- Raw egg, as this can impair absorption
- Single biotin supplements should not be taken long term unless combined with a B complex

Folate

The Snapshot

Folate is involved in many fundamental biological processes including synthesis and repair of our DNA. For this reason it is essential during pregnancy for proper growth and development. A healthy heart relies on adequate folate and as a member of the B vitamin family it also helps release energy from fuel (food) to keep our motor running!

Supplementation is recommended during pregnancy. It is especially important during the first four weeks of pregnancy for development of the neural tube. Even if following a healthy diet, the body can absorb folate better in supplemental form than from food. Supplementation can also be beneficial for those with risk factors for heart disease and alongside iron for those with low iron or anaemia.

The terms folate and folic acid are often used interchangeably, however folate is the nutrient used by the body and folic acid is the synthesised supplemental source. Up to 50% of the population may lack the ability to properly convert folic acid to folate.

Calcium folinate/folinic acid is the preferred supplemental source, especially in pregnancy, as it has been shown to increase folate levels more efficiently and effectively than folic acid supplements.

Other names

Vitamin B9

What does it do?

Folate is required for the synthesis and repair of our DNA and is involved in many fundamental biological processes in the body. It is therefore particularly important in times of rapid development and growth. It's required alongside iron, vitamins B6 and B12 for the production of healthy red blood cells and alongside vitamin B12 and vitamin B6 to help reduce homocysteine levels. Homocysteine is an amino acid, excess amounts of which can damage artery walls and increase the risk of blood clots. High homocysteine levels are a risk factor in cardiovascular disease.

One of the most well known roles of folate is in pregnancy. Folate is vital for proper development of an infant's neural tube, from which the brain and spinal cord develop. Once developed, the neural tube closes to encase and protect the brain and spinal cord. This process begins and is generally complete by week five of pregnancy, before most women even know they are pregnant. Therefore it's vital that women maintain healthy levels of folate prior to conception and during the first four weeks of pregnancy. Healthy folate levels can also help improve chances of conception.

As with the other B vitamins, folate is involved in the release of energy from food, forming an essential part of our metabolic 'spark plug' converting our fuel (food) into active energy to keep our motor running!

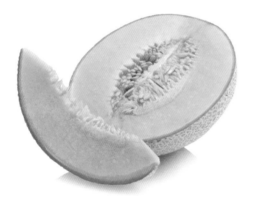

How do I know if I'm deficient?

Folate is a relatively common deficiency. It is highly sensitive to heat, air and light and is therefore easily destroyed from our food. There are also common genetic polymorphisms which can hinder some people's ability to absorb and metabolise the common supplemental source, folic acid. These polymorphisms affect around 50% of the population. Deficiency symptoms can be very subtle and vague and can easily go undiagnosed.

Signs and Symtoms

MILD DEFICIENCY
- Weakness/fatigue
- Irritability
- Headaches
- Loss of appetite

SEVERE DEFICIENCY
- Anaemia
- Low birth weight, premature birth and neural tube defects (during pregnancy)

What foods does it come in?

Asparagus	Lima beans	Sweet potato	Oranges
Brussels sprouts	Soy beans	Broccoli	Orange juice
Spinach	Lentils	Green leafy vegetables	Oatmeal
Romaine lettuce	Liver	Sprouts	Wheat germ
Beans	Peas	Cantaloupe	Yeast

How much should I have?

	AI	UL
INFANTS		
0 – 6 months	65mcg/day	Not possible to establish
7 – 12 months	80mcg/day	Not possible to establish

	RDI	UL
TODDLERS		
1 – 3 years	150mcg/day	300mcg/day
4 – 8 years	200mcg/day	400mcg/day

	RDI	UL
CHILDREN		
Boys 9 – 13 years	300mcg/day	6000mcg/day
Boys 14 – 18 years	400mcg/day	800mcg/day
Girls 9 – 13 years	300mcg/day	600mcg/day
Girls 14 – 18 years	400mcg/day	800mcg/day

	RDI	UL
ADULTS		
Men 19 – 70 + years	400mcg/day	1000mcg/day
Women 19 – 70 years	400mcg/day	10000mg/day

	RDI	UL
PREGNANCY		
14 – 18 years	600mcg/day	800mcg/day
18 – 50 years	600mcg/day	1000mcg/day

	RDI	UL
LACTATION		
14 – 18 years	600mcg/day	800mcg/day
18 – 50 years	600mcg/day	1000mcg/day

THERAPEUTIC ADULT DOSE

400 - 500mcg/day is the recommended dose for all women of childbearing age.
400 - 500mcg/day is also recommended for those with cardiovascular risk factors or low iron levels.

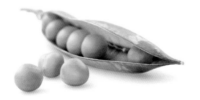

Is a supplement recommended for me?

Folate supplements are recommended for all women of child bearing age, particularly during conception and pregnancy, as birth defects generally occur in the very early stages of pregnancy when the neural tube is forming. Supplementation can also be beneficial for those with cardiovascular risk factors or alongside iron for healthy blood.

Which supplement should I choose?

Folic acid and calcium folinate/folinic acid are the supplemental sources of folate, with calcium folinate/folinic acid providing the best absorption. As with other B vitamins; folate is best taken alongside the B complex family. If supplementing for conception and pregnancy, a specific pregnancy multivitamin and mineral supplement containing 500mg of calcium folinate is ideal.

When should I take my supplement?

As with all B vitamins; folate is best taken with food. As B vitamins are part of our metabolic 'spark plug', helping to support energy production. They are best taken in the morning to avoid possible sleep disturbance, unless you're planning big night out where that extra energy boost could come in handy!

What happens if I take too much?

Doses above the recommended UL are generally not detrimental; however prolonged high doses have been associated with adverse reproductive and developmental effects and have been linked to some forms of cancer, although a definite link is inconclusive. For those with B12 deficiency, high intake of folate can exacerbate the deficiency and affect neurological symptoms.

Matching it up

TAKE FOLATE WITH

- B complex
- B12 is required for the metabolism and absorption of folic acid
- B12 and B6 to help reduce homocysteine
- Iron, B6 and B12 to treat anaemia and low Iron levels

DON'T TAKE FOLATE WITH

- Single folate supplements should not be taken long term unless combined with a B complex

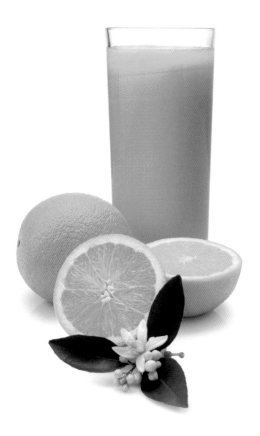

Vitamin B12

The Snapshot

As a member of the B vitamin family, B12 assists the conversion of fuel (food) to energy to keep our motor running! It also supports a healthy nervous system, mood and stress response. Vitamin B12 is essential for maintenance of a healthy heart and blood cells and is also required alongside folate for the production of cellular DNA.

As vitamin B12 is mainly found in animal sources, vegetarians can often benefit from supplementation. Those with cardiovascular risk factors can also benefit from B12 supplementation alongside folate and B6.

Cobalamin is the naturally occurring form found in food, while cyanocobalamin is the form most commonly found in supplements and hydroxocobalamin is the form most commonly found in B12 injections.

Other names

Cobalamin, cyanocobalamin, hydroxocobalamin

What does it do?

Vitamin B12 is involved in the metabolism of all cells and is required, in combination with folate, for the production of DNA. As with the other members of the B vitamin group, it plays a key role in the release of energy from food and is essential for the production of neurotransmitters which effect mood and support healthy functioning of the nervous system.

Vitamin B12 works with folate and vitamin B6 to help reduce homocysteine levels by metabolising it into a safer form, which can be actively used by the body. Homocysteine is an amino acid, excess amounts of which can damage artery walls and increase risk of blood clots. High homocysteine levels have been shown to be a risk factor in cardiovascular disease.

Vitamin B12 is also required for the manufacture of healthy blood cells.

How do I know if I'm deficient?

Most people have the ability to store many years worth of vitamin B12 in the liver to prevent deficiency, even when dietary intake may be inadequate for extended periods. Therefore severe deficiency is not common in the average person. Deficiency is generally related to an inherited lack of intrinsic factor.

Intrinsic factor is kind of like B12's GPS. It helps direct vitamin B12 from the stomach to the bloodstream and cells where is can be used. For those lacking this vital factor, B12 can't navigate its way to the bloodstream meaning that most oral forms of vitamin B12 are excreted rather than absorbed, therefore vitamin B12 injections may be required to bypass the digestive system.

Good stomach acid is also essential for the breakdown and absorption of oral vitamin B12, therefore the elderly who often have decreased stomach acid, can be at higher risk of deficiency.

The clinical presentation of vitamin B12 deficiency is pernicious anaemia. Symptoms include low energy/fatigue, pale skin, irritability, depression, tingling hands and feet and inability to focus/concentrate. If left untreated, this deficiency disease can lead to irreversible neurological and nerve damage, even once the underlying deficiency has been corrected. The longer the condition remains untreated, the less likely the chance of complete symptom reversal.

Signs and Symtoms

MILD DEFICIENCY
- Low mood/depression
- Low energy
- Poor memory/concentration
- Irritability

SEVERE DEFICIENCY
- Pernicious anaemia

Is a supplement recommended for me?

Those with a lack of intrinsic factor to metabolise vitamin B12 will require supplementation, often in the form of injections. However, therapeutic oral supplementation in doses of 1000-2000mg per day can be effective in some cases. As vitamin B12 is mainly found in animal sources, vegetarians can often benefit from supplementation.

What foods does it come in?

Liver	Kidney	Salmon	Cottage cheese
Trout	Crab	Sardines	Cheese
Beef	Oysters	Veal	Eggs
Clams	Lamb	Milk	
Brains	Tuna	Yoghurt	

How much should I have?

INFANTS	AI	
0 – 6 months	0.4mcg/day	
7 – 12 months	0.5mcg/day	
TODDLERS	RDI	
1 – 3 years	0.7mcg/day	
4 – 8 years	1mcg/day	
CHILDREN	RDI	
Boys 9 – 13 years	1.8mcg/day	
Boys 14 – 18 years	2.4mcg/day	
Girls 9 – 13 years	1.8mcg/day	
Girls 14 – 18 years	2.4mcg/day	
ADULTS	RDI	
Men 19 – 70 + years	2.4mcg/day	
Women 19 – 70 + years	2.4mcg/day	
PREGNANCY	RDI	
14 + years	2.6mcg/day	
LACTATION	RDI	
14 + years	2.8mcg/day	

THERAPEUTIC ADULT DOSE

50 – 100mcg/day is a good dose to support heart health and help improve energy.
1000mcg – 2000mcg/day is recommended to treat deficiency.
There is no recommended upper limit (UL) for vitamin B12.

Matching it up

TAKE VITAMIN B12 WITH
- B12 is required for metabolism and absorption of folic acid
- B complex

DON'T TAKE VITAMIN B12 WITH
- Single B12 supplements should not be taken long term unless combined with a B complex

Which supplement should I choose?

Unlike most vitamins and minerals, absorption of vitamin B12 actually begins in the mouth. Therefore some people lacking intrinsic factor report benefits from sublingual supplements, however this is yet to be clinically proven. Otherwise, most supplements come in tablets in the form of cyanocobalamin. This is best taken in conjunction with the other members of the B vitamin family.

When should I take my supplement?

As with all B vitamins; vitamin B12 is best taken with food. With the involvement of the B vitamins in energy production they are also best taken in the morning to avoid possible sleep disturbance.

What happens if I take too much?

As vitamin B12 is water soluble, any excess can be easily excreted from the body; therefore vitamin B12 is extremely safe and doesn't appear to have any toxic side effects even in large doses.

Choline

The Snapshot

Although our body can produce small amounts of choline, it is considered an essential nutrient as dietary sources are required to supply sufficient amounts to maintain health. Choline is essential for the structure and function of all cell membranes. It is vital for optimal brain and memory function and adequate intake is essential during pregnancy and breastfeeding for healthy development of the brain and neural tube.

Choline is important for heart health and possesses mild anti-inflammatory properties. It also acts like a GPS for nerve signals and fat transport, helping the nervous system send vital signals to the muscles and helping to transport fat from the liver to cells where it is required.

Supplementation is highly recommended during pregnancy and breastfeeding to assist in the prevention of birth defects and support optimal brain development. Supplements can also be of benefit for those with cardiovascular risk factors.

Choline supplements are available in the form of lecithin, which provides phosphatidylcholine, or in multivitamins in the form of choline bitartrate or choline chloride.

Other names

Choline is not known by any other name.

What does it do?

Choline is involved in the synthesis of the fat containing building blocks of all cell membranes. These components are responsible for ensuring cell membrane integrity, flexibility and function, including the absorption of nutrients and communication between cells. Choline is a major component of acetylcholine. Acetylcholine is the major neurotransmitter involved in sending signals between nerves and muscles. Our body's own GPS, for directing nerve signals to the muscles they need to activate! Basically, choline helps keep cell walls healthy and functioning at their best, protecting them and allowing them to 'chat' between themselves!

Choline is essential for optimal foetal brain and neural tube development during pregnancy. The amount of choline present in the mother's diet during pregnancy reduces the risk of neural tube defects and may influence brain health and lifelong learning and memory capacity of the infant. It's also essential during breastfeeding to support the rapid brain development. Adequate levels are also vital later in life to maintain healthy brain function and assist in the prevention of age related memory loss, as long as you remember to take it!

Phosphatidylcholine is required in the transport of fat from the liver to cells where it's required. Impairment of this transport mechanism can lead to a build up of fat in the liver.

Choline and its metabolite betaine have been shown to possess anti-inflammatory properties. Betaine, metabolised from choline can also assist in the conversion of homocysteine to methionine, reducing homocysteine levels, which can damage artery walls and increase the risk of blood clots.

How do I know if I'm deficient?

Research has shown that around 90% of the general population are not reaching their Adequate Intake (AI) of choline. This is of particular concern for pregnant women, with deficiency associated with brain development and birth defects. Those with a high alcohol consumption level are also at increased risk as alcohol can deplete choline levels.

Signs and Symtoms

MILD DEFICIENCY
- Fatigue
- Insomnia
- Poor memory
- Impaired nerve and muscle function
- Possible impairment of foetal growth and development (pregnancy)

SEVERE DEFICIENCY
- Birth defects, failure to thrive (pregnancy)
- Fatty Liver/liver dysfunction
- Risk factor for cardiovascular disease

What foods does it come in?

Lecithin granules	Milk	Spinach	Kidney beans
Egg yolk	Peanuts	Bananas	Corn
Beef liver	Almonds	Oranges	Quinoa
Chicken	Potatoes	Lentils	Amaranth
Soybeans	Tomatoes	Oats	Wheat germ
Tofu	Cauliflower	Barley	Sesame seeds
			Flaxseeds

How much should I have?

INFANTS	AI	UL
0 – 6 months	125mg/day	Not possible to establish
7 – 12 months	150mg/day	Not possible to establish
TODDLERS	**AI**	**UL**
1 – 3 years	200 mg/day	1000mg/day
4 – 8 years	250mg/day	1000mg/day
CHILDREN	**AI**	**UL**
Boys 9 – 13 years	375mg/day	1000mg/day
Boys 14 – 18 years	550mg/day	3000mg/day
Girls 9 – 13 years	375mg/day	1000mg/day
Girls 14 – 18 years	400mg/day	3000mg/day
ADULTS	**AI**	**UL**
Men 19 – 70 + years	550mg/day	3500mg/day
Women 19 – 70 + years	425mg/day	3500mg/day
PREGNANCY	**AI**	**UL**
14 – 18 years	415mg/day	3000mg/day
18 – 50 years	440mg/day	3500mg/day
LACTATION	**AI**	**UL**
14 – 18 years	525mg/day	3000mg/day
18 – 50 years	550mg/day	3500mg/day

THERAPEUTIC ADULT DOSE

400 - 600mg/day is generally sufficient to support brain and cardiovascular health.
500mg is ideal during pregnancy to support healthy brain development and assist in the prevention of neural tube defects.
There is no recommended daily intake (RDI) for choline. Recommendations are based on the adequate intake (AI).

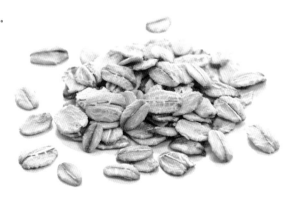

Is a supplement recommended for me?

Supplementation is recommended during pregnancy to help prevent birth defects and support healthy foetal growth and brain development. Choline supplements may also be beneficial later in life to help support memory and brain health. Those with cardiovascular risk factors may also benefit from supplementation.

Which supplement should I choose?

Choline is found mainly as a component of multivitamins in the forms of choline bitatrate or choline chloride, which provide the highest levels of choline. Phosphatidylcholine is derived from lecithin. Lecithin supplements provide phosphatidylcholine at levels anywhere between 20-90% depending on the quality of the supplement. The exact amount of phosphatidylcholine in the lecithin supplement should be stipulated on the label.

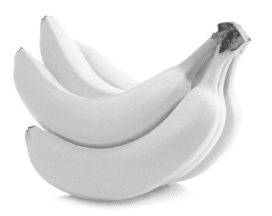

Matching it up

TAKE CHOLINE WITH

- Choline can be beneficial in conjunction with vitamins B6, B12 and folate for reduction of homocysteine levels and improved heart health
- Choline is beneficial in conjunction with folate to support growth and reduce the risk of neural tube defects in pregnancy

DON'T TAKE CHOLINE WITH

- No interactions noted

When should I take my supplement?

Choline is best taken with or just before food, preferably early in the day as it may disrupt sleep.

What happens if I take too much?

Doses of 7,500mg/day have been associated with a slight decrease in blood pressure which could cause light-headedness/dizziness. Doses above 10,000mg have been associated with a 'fishy' odour; increased sweating, increased salivation and vomiting. The odour is caused by an increased excretion of trimethylamine, which is a metabolite of choline. However, choline is non toxic and these side effects are easily reversed when intake is decreased.

Vitamin C

The Snapshot

Vitamin C is one of our bodyguard nutrients, helping to protect our body by supporting a healthy immune system and acting as a potent antioxidant, to help ward off the effects of environmental damage and aging. Vitamin C is also involved in the production of collagen and is often included in beauty creams and treatments.

Supplements are available in the form of ascorbic acid, calcium ascorbate and sodium ascorbate, or a combination of these. Ascorbic acid is the purest form of vitamin C, however calcium and sodium ascorbate are less acidic and can therefore be gentler on the stomach. Supplementation is recommended during times of cold/flu, infection, weakened immune system or wound healing. Supplements can also be beneficial to support healthy skin and provide antioxidant protection against cellular damage and signs of aging.

Other names

Ascorbic acid, calcium ascorbate, sodium ascorbate

What does it do?

Vitamin C is involved in white blood cell activity and antibody production, which helps the body fight infection. Vitamin C helps provide the artillery our white blood cells need to keep them primed and ready to fight off any pending attack!

Vitamin C is an integral nutrient in the production of collagen. Collagen forms the basis of all our connective tissue, which connects and helps protect our bones, muscles and all our internal organs. Collagen is a main component of our skin, teeth, bones, cartilage, ligaments and tendons and is vital for wound healing. Collagen can also help keep our skin 'plump' and 'firm'. A good vitamin C supplement is a great inexpensive way to help boost collagen without the price tag of expensive beauty creams!

Vitamin C is a powerful water soluble antioxidant, protecting the body from harmful oxidative damage, which can lead to increased signs of ageing and disease.

How do I know if I'm deficient?

Severe vitamin C deficiency is uncommon in developed countries and leads to a condition known as scurvy. Symptoms of scurvy relate to the reduced collagen production and include brown/red splotches on the skin due to broken capillaries, bleeding mouth and gums, loss of teeth, reduced wound healing and ultimately death if left untreated.

MILD DEFICIENCY

- Reduced resistance to infection
- Reduced recovery and wound healing
- Reduced fertility (particularly in smokers)

SEVERE DEFICIENCY

- Scurvy

What foods does it come in?

Kiwi fruit	Strawberries	Guava	Brussels sprouts
Orange	Cranberries	Paw paw	Parsley
Orange juice	Cranberry juice	Grapes	Potato
Cantaloupe	Tomato	Raspberries	Sweet potato
Grapefruit	Tomato juice	Green pepper	Cabbage
Grapefruit juice	Watermelon	Cauliflower	
Blackcurrants	Pineapple	Broccoli	

Is a supplement recommended for me?

Supplementation is recommended during times of cold/flu, infection, weakened immune system or wound healing to help support recovery.

Which supplement should I choose?

Supplements generally contain vitamin C in the form of ascorbic acid, calcium ascorbate, sodium ascorbate or a combination of these. Ascorbic acid is the pure form of vitamin C. The 'buffered' mineral ascorbates, calcium ascorbate and sodium ascorbate are less acidic and are therefore gentler on the stomach.

Some vitamin C supplements also contain bioflavonoids. Bioflavonoids occur naturally with vitamin C in foods, for example they can be found in the pith of citrus fruits, and can help increase the activity of vitamin C in the body.

Vitamin C is available in chewable, powder and tablet form. There are no discernible differences between absorption rates of the various supplementation options, the key is to look at the amount and type of vitamin C the supplement is providing, the rest is personal preference.

How much should I have?

	AI
INFANTS	
0 – 6 months	25mg/day
7 – 12 months	30mg/day

	RDI
TODDLERS	
1 – 3 years	35mg/day
4 – 8 years	35mg/day

	RDI
CHILDREN	
Boys 9 – 13 years	40mg/day
Boys 14 – 18 years	40mg/day
Girls 9 – 13 years	40mg/day
Girls 14 – 18 years	40mg/day

	RDI
ADULTS	
Men 19 – 70 + years	45mg/day
Women 19 – 70 + years	45mg/day

	RDI
PREGNANCY	
14 – 18 years	55mg/day
19 – 50 years	60mg/day

	RDI
LACTATION	
14 + 18 years	80mg/day
19 – 50 years	85mg/day

50 - 1000mg/day is a good dose to assist in the maintenance of a healthy immune system, mild antioxidant activity and collagen support.
1000 - 5000mg + /day is recommended to assist in the treatment of cold and flu, other acute infections and wound healing as well as antioxidant activity. This is best divided into smaller doses over the day to avoid digestive disturbance.
There is no recommended upper limit (UL) for vitamin C.

Matching it up

TAKE VITAMIN C WITH
- Bioflavonoids can help increase the activity of vitamin C in the body
- Vitamin C is beneficial in combination with vitamin A, vitamin E and zinc for the treatment and prevention of macular degeneration

DON'T TAKE VITAMIN C WITH
- No interactions noted

When should I take my supplement?

Vitamin C can be taken at any time of day with or without food.

What happens if I take too much?

Vitamin C is water soluble and easily excreted from the body, it therefore has no toxicity. However, excess consumption can lead to digestive discomfort and diarrhoea as the body excretes the excess.

During times of cold/flu, infection or weakened immunity the demand for vitamin C increases and therefore digestive tolerance of vitamin C can increase dramatically. During these times it can be beneficial to consume consistent divided doses of vitamin C until you feel a slight 'rumbling' in the stomach to indicate that tolerance has been reached, providing you with your maximum intake and maximum immune support.

Vitamin D

The Snapshot

Vitamin D is commonly recognised as the 'sunshine' vitamin, as we can obtain vitamin D from exposure to the sun.

Adequate vitamin D levels are particularly important for bone health, hormone activity and during pregnancy for healthy foetal development. Low levels are associated with mood and depression.

The elderly are at greater risk of vitamin D deficiency, especially those in nursing homes or housebound with little sun exposure. It's also important for pregnant women to ensure adequate vitamin D to support the health of both mother and baby.

Supplements are best taken in the form of vitamin D3, which is better absorbed than vitamin D2.

Other names

Ergocalciferol (vitamin D2), cholecalciferol (vitamin D3)

What does it do?

Vitamin D is essential for the absorption of calcium and the maintenance of bone health. It helps transport calcium to our bones to help maintain optimal bone strength.

Vitamin D is actually known as a pro-hormone as it can be converted into an active hormone, which accounts for much of its widespread activity in the body.

Adequate levels are vital for fertility and conception and vitamin D continues to be important during pregnancy and breastfeeding for formation of the baby's bones and teeth. Low levels during pregnancy are linked to low birth weight, growth retardation and premature labour. More recently, lack of vitamin D during pregnancy has been associated with a range of other disorders in the child, including type 1 diabetes, Multiple sclerosis, manic depression, anxiety and schizophrenia. Low levels can also affect the health of the mother, increasing the risk of pre-eclampsia, gestational diabetes and infection. So ensuring adequate levels during pregnancy is vital.

How do I know if I'm deficient?

Vitamin D deficiency is increasingly common, particularly due to the increased use of sunscreen and increased time spent indoors. Severe vitamin D deficiency results in a condition known as osteomalacia in adults or rickets in children. These conditions are characterised by a softening/weakening of the bones. In children this can lead to the malformation of bones or bones bending under the weight of the body. In adults it can lead to stress fractures, bone pain and muscle weakness.

Signs and Symtoms

MILD DEFICIENCY
- Increased bone loss
- Decreased bone mineral density
- Low Mood/depression

SEVERE DEFICIENCY
- Osteomalacia (adults)/rickets (children)

What foods does it come in?

Milk	Tuna	Herring liver oil	Chicken liver
Butter	Cod liver oil	Prawns	Egg yolk
Salmon	Halibut liver oil	Beef liver	Sprouted seeds

Is a supplement recommended for me?

Due to the risks associated with excess sun exposure, vitamin D supplements are considered a preferable method of ensuring adequate vitamin D levels in some people. Supplementation is highly recommended for the elderly, particularly those who may be house bound or in nursing homes. Supplementation is also advised in pregnant women to ensure adequate levels for proper foetal development. Vitamin D supplements may also be useful for those suffering low mood or the 'winter blues' as lack of vitamin D can exacerbate melancholy and depression.

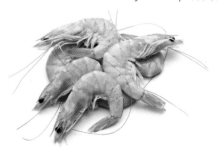

Which supplement should I choose?

You should look for a supplement containing vitamin D3, which is better absorbed than vitamin D2.

When should I take my supplement?

As a fat soluble nutrient, vitamin D is best taken with food.

Matching it up

TAKE VITAMIN D WITH
- Can be taken alone

DON'T TAKE VITAMIN D WITH
- No known interactions

How much should I have?

1 International Unit (IU) of Vitamin D is equivalent to 0.025mcg

	AI	UL
INFANTS		
0 - 6 months	5mcg/day (200IU)	25mcg (1000IU)
7 - 12 months	5mcg/day (200IU)	25mcg (1000IU)
TODDLERS	RDI	UL
1 - 3 years	5mcg/day (200IU)	80mcg/day (3200IU)
4 - 8 years	5mcg/day (200IU)	80mcg/day (3200IU)
CHILDREN	RDI	UL
Boys 9 - 13 years	5mcg/day (200IU)	80mcg/day (3200IU)
Boys 14 - 18 years	5mcg/day (200IU)	80mcg/day (3200IU)
Girls 9 - 13 years	5mcg/day (200IU)	80mcg/day (3200IU)
Girls 14 - 18 years	5mcg/day (200IU)	80mcg/day (3200IU)
ADULTS	RDI	UL
Men 19 - 50 years	5mcg/day (200IU)	80mcg/day (3200IU)
Men 50 - 70 years	10mcg/day (400IU)	80mcg/day (3200IU)
Men 70 + years	15mcg/day (600IU)	80mcg/day (3200IU)
Women 19 - 50 years	5mcg/day (200IU)	80mcg/day (3200IU)
Women 50 - 70 years	10mcg/day (400IU)	80mcg/day (3200IU)
Women 70 + years	15mcg/day (600IU)	80mcg/day (3200IU)
PREGNANCY	RDI	UL
14 + years	15mcg/day (600IU)	80mcg/day (3200IU)
LACTATION	RDI	UL
14 + years	15mcg/day (600IU)	80mcg/day (3200IU)

THERAPEUTIC ADULT DOSE

25mcg (1000IU)/day is the recommended therapeutic dose to help correct and prevent deficiency.

Up to 100mcg - 400mcg (5000IU - 20000IU) may be required to correct significant deficiency, however these higher doses should only be taken under the guidance of a health care professional.

What happens if I take too much?

Vitamin D toxicity is very rare, however excess vitamin D can cause symptoms such as nausea, digestive upset, diarrhoea and fatigue. It can also cause calcium to build up in the bloodstream, which can affect the nervous and cardiovascular systems.

Vitamin E

The Snapshot

Vitamin E is another one of our bodyguard antioxidant nutrients, helping to protect cells from the effects of aging and environmental damage.

Supplements can be beneficial for smokers and those exposed to environments pollutants, and to support heart health, improve fertility and assist in the prevention of macular degeneration.

Most vitamin E supplements come in the form of d-alphatocopherol and dl-alphatocophaerol. D-alpha tocopherol is the most natural form and is the best supplement to choose for optimal absorption. Some high quality supplements also contain vitamin E in the form of tocotrienols, which have the most potent antioxidant activity.

Vitamin E can be absorbed through the skin and is often found in cosmetic and therapeutic skin creams.

Other names

D-alpha tocopherol, dl-alpha tocopherol, tocotrienols

What does it do?

Vitamin E is a potent fat soluble antioxidant, acting as one of our cellular bodyguards to protect cells against free radical damage. In this role it can help reduce the effects of aging and assist in cancer prevention.

Vitamin E is essential for eye health, helping support development of the retina and protect against oxidative damage. It also protects the vitamin A molecule from damage, which is important for eye health, and can help prevent macular degeneration, especially in combination with vitamin A, vitamin C and zinc.

Vitamin E has been shown to be beneficial in helping maintain overall cardiovascular health for a number of reasons. It can help reduce the risk of blood clots, reduce the risk of atherosclerosis and may assist in the reduction of cholesterol as well as the oxidation of 'bad' LDL cholesterol.

Vitamin E may help improve male fertility by protecting sperm from oxidative damage and improving sperm function and motility.

How do I know if I'm deficient?

Vitamin E deficiency is extremely rare. It is generally caused by secondary metabolic disorders affecting absorption of vitamin E and rarely from lack of vitamin E in the diet.

Is a supplement recommended for me?

Supplementation can be beneficial for those exposed to increased oxidative stress, such as smokers. It may also assist those with cardiovascular risk factors and help treat and prevent macular degeneration, particularly in combination with nutrients vitamin A, vitamin C and zinc.

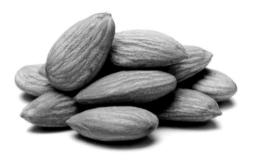

Which supplement should I choose?

Most supplements contain vitamin E in the form of alpha tocopherol as this is the most widely studied and well absorbed. Alpha tocopherol is available in two forms, d-alpha tocopherol and dl-alpha tocopherol. D-alpha tocopherol is the most natural form and has the highest bioavailability. Therefore you should look for d-alphatocopherol when choosing a supplement.

The lesser known tocotrienols are also gaining in popularity. Tocotrienols have a more potent antioxidant activity than the tocopherols and many high quality supplements contain tocotrienols in combination with d-alpha tocopherol.

What foods does it come in?

Apricot oil	Margarine	Cashews	Wheat germ
Safflower oil	Sunflower seeds	Sweet potato	Wholegrain bread
Sunflower oil	Almonds	Asparagus	Crab meat
Egg yolk	Peanuts	Spinach	Prawns
			Fish

How much should I have?

IU is often used when referring to measurements of fat soluble nutrients vitamin A, vitamin D, vitamin K or vitamin E. The below references are given in terms of natural vitamin E.

1mg of natural vitamin E (d-alpha tocopherol) is approximately equivalent to 1.5IU.
1mg of synthesised vitamin E (dl-alpha tocopherol) is approximately equivalent to 1IU.

INFANTS	AI	UL
0 - 6 months	4mg/day (6IU)	Not possible to establish
7 - 12 months	5mg/day (7.5IU)	Not possible to establish
TODDLERS	RDI	UL
1 - 3 years	5mg/day (7.5IU)	70mg/day (105IU)
4 - 8 years	6mg/day (9IU)	100mg/day (150IU)
CHILDREN	RDI	UL
Boys 9 - 13 years	9mg/day (13.5IU)	180mg/day (270IU)
Boys 14 - 18 years	10mg/day (15IU)	250mg/day (375IU)
Girls 9 - 13 years	8mg/day (12IU)	180mg/day (270IU)
Girls 14 - 18 years	8mg/day (12IU)	250mg/day (375IU)
ADULTS	RDI	UL
Men 19 - 70 + years	10mg/day (15IU)	300mg/day (450IU)
Women 19 - 70 + years	7mg/day (10.5IU)	300mg/day (450IU)
PREGNANCY	RDI	UL
14 - 18 years	7mg/day (10.5IU)	300mg/day (450IU)
19 + years	8mg/day (12IU)	300mg/day (450IU)
LACTATION	RDI	UL
14 - 18 years	12mg/day (18IU)	300mg/day (450IU)
19 + years	11mg/day (16.5IU)	300mg/day (450IU)

THERAPEUTIC ADULT DOSE

67mg - 133mg/day (100 - 200IU) is a good dose for general health and antioxidant activity.
133mg - 266mg/day (200IU - 400IU) is recommended for cardiovascular health.
266mg - 533mg (400IU - 800IU) can be beneficial in some cases but should only be taken under advisement of your health care professional.

Matching it up

TAKE VITAMIN E WITH

- Vitamin E is beneficial in combination with vitamin A, vitamin C and zinc in the treatment and prevention of macular degeneration
- Vitamin C, vitamin B3, glutathione and selenium are required to keep vitamin E biologically active in the body

DON'T TAKE VITAMIN E WITH

- As vitamin E can thin the blood it can interact with warfarin and should only be taken under advisement from your health care professional

When should I take my supplement?

As a fat soluble nutrient, vitamin E is best taken with food.

What happens if I take too much?

Excessive doses of supplemental vitamin E can interfere with vitamin K and disrupt the blood's ability to clot, leading to increased risk of haemorrhage. Supplemental doses should not exceed 1000mg (1500IU) unless advised by a health care professional.

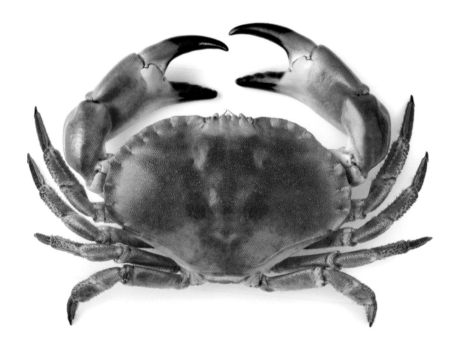

Minerals

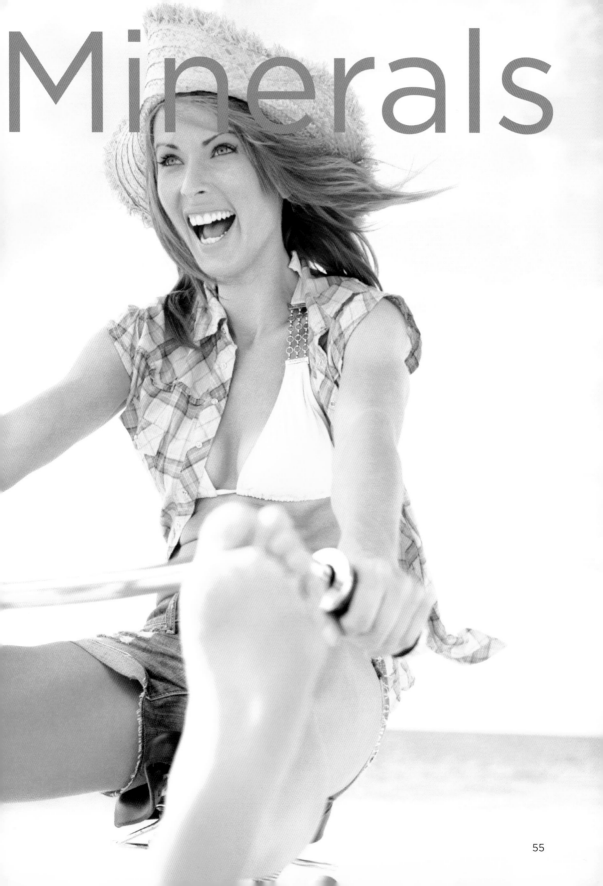

Calcium

The Snapshot

Calcium is widely known as our bone health nutrient. Around 99% of the calcium in our body is stored in our bones and teeth where it helps support growth, strength, regeneration and repair. Calcium, in conjunction with magnesium, also plays a role in muscle contraction and relaxation as well as the transmission of nerve impulses.

Those with low dietary calcium intake or who are at risk of osteoporosis may benefit from supplementation. Supplements are commonly available in the form of calcium carbonate, calcium citrate and calcium hydroxyapatite. Citrate and hydroxyapatite form are the best sources to look for in a supplement, alongside vitamin D to aid absorption.

Other names

Calcium is not known by any other name.

What does it do?

Calcium is essential for bone health. Most of the calcium in our body (up to 99%) is stored in our bones and teeth. Although bones appear as a stable, solid structure, our bones are alive! The bone matrix is constantly being broken down and new bone regenerated in its place to maintain bone health and strength. Calcium is a vital link in this regeneration process.

Before the age of 20, bone growth is more rapid than breakdown. In the early 20s peak bone mass is achieved, with men reaching a higher peak bone mass than women. During our 20s and 30s the bone renewal cycle becomes balanced. The stronger the bones are at this point, the longer they will keep their strength. Around the age of 35, bones begin to break down faster than they rebuild. Overall, women lose approximately one third of their bone mineral density between menopause and the age of 80. This is because estrogen has a protective effect on the bones and once this begins to decline we are at greater risk of osteoporosis. Consuming adequate levels of calcium can slow the process of osteoporosis by at least 30 – 50%.

Calcium is also important in combination with magnesium for muscle contraction and relaxation. Calcium is required to activate nerve cells, which then send signals to stimulate and activate our muscles as required. Magnesium works in opposition, to prevent excess calcium activating nerve cells, which can cause excess muscle stimulation and cramping. Adequate calcium to magnesium balance helps maintain muscles in a relaxed state, preventing cramps, twitches and tension.

Calcium is also involved in the release of neurotransmitters including serotonin and dopamine, which affect mood and stress response.

How do I know if I'm deficient?

With the average diet containing less than 50% of calcium requirements, mild deficiency is relatively common. Diets high in protein can also lead to increased calcium loss from the bones. This increases the demand for calcium, yet high protein diets are often lacking this nutrient, so those following a high protein diet can be at higher risk of deficiency. Diets high in sodium (salt) can also increase calcium excretion, as can excess caffeine and alcohol consumption. Unfortunately salt, caffeine and alcohol are all common additions to today's fast paced lifestyle!

Calcium deficiency has no immediate effects on the body and can therefore often go undiagnosed until more permanent damage has already been done. It's important not to wait until symptoms arise before topping up your calcium intake!

Signs and Symtoms

MILD DEFICIENCY
- Increased bone loss, usually without the presence of any noticeable signs and symptoms

SEVERE DEFICIENCY
- Hypocalemia: Symptoms include numbness, tingling fingers, cramps, fatigue, poor appetite and disturbed heart rhythm

What foods does it come in?

Dairy products	Sesame seeds	Spinach	Soy milk
Seaweed	Molasses	Chinese cabbage	Quinoa
Kelp	Broccoli	Oranges	Small amounts in
Sardines	Green beans	Figs	most grains
Almonds			

How much should I have?

	AI	UL
INFANTS		
0 – 6 months	210mg/day	Not possible to establish
7 – 12 months	270mg/day	Not possible to establish
TODDLERS	RDI	UL
1 – 3 years	500mg/day	2500mg/day
4 – 8 years	700mg/day	2500mg/day
CHILDREN	RDI	UL
Boys 9 – 11 years	1000mg/day	2500mg/day
Boys 12 – 18 years	1300mg/day	2500mg/day
Girls 9 – 11 years	1000mg/day	2500mg/day
Girls 12 – 18 years	1300mg/day	2500mg/day
ADULTS	RDI	UL
Men 19 – 70 years	1000mg/day	2500mg/day
Men 70 + years	1300mg/day	2500mg/day
Women 19 – 70 years	1000mg/day	2500mg/day
Women 70 + years	1300mg/day	2500mg/day
PREGNANCY	RDI	UL
14 – 18 years	1300mg/day	2500mg/day
19 – 50 years	1000mg/day	2500mg/day
LACTATION	RDI	UL
14 – 18 years	1300mg/day	2500mg/day
19 + years	1000mg/day	2500mg/day

THERAPEUTIC ADULT DOSE

1000 - 1500mg/day is the recommended therapeutic dose unless otherwise advised by your health care professional.

Is a supplement recommended for me?

Calcium supplements are particularly beneficial for post menopausal women, the elderly and during pregnancy when demand increases. Supplementary calcium can also benefit those following high protein diets or indulging in a little too much salt, caffeine or alcohol!

Our ability to absorb calcium from either food or supplements decreases as we age. Infants and young children are able to absorb up to 60% of the calcium they ingest to support their rapid growth. This decreases to around 15-20% as we reach adulthood and continues to decrease the older we get, therefore supplemental doses of calcium become more important as we age.

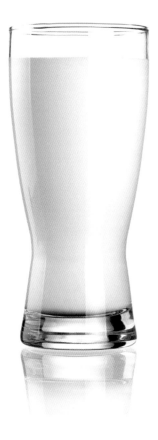

Which supplement should I choose?

Calcium is available in the form of calcium carbonate, calcium citrate, calcium phosphate, calcium gluconate and calcium hydroxyapatite. Supplements most commonly contain calcium in the form of carbonate, citrate or hydroxyapatite.

Calcium carbonate is the cheapest and most common source of calcium and provides a high dose of elemental calcium (around 40%). However, calcium carbonate is the substance chalk is made from and is used in manufacturing to make cement, lime stone and mortar as well as some antacid preparations. As such, it is more difficult for the body to absorb, requiring a good acidic gastric environment to sufficiently break it down for absorption. This can be particularly troublesome for the elderly who generally have reduced gastric acid; therefore calcium carbonate commonly causes side effects such as constipation, bloating and excess gas in these people. The presence of carbonate in the gut can also decrease the ability to absorb other nutrients.

Calcium citrate provides a lower dose of elemental calcium (around 21%), however it has been shown to have a higher absorption rate (around 25% higher) than a carbonate and is not linked with any side effects. It is therefore a preferable supplemental form.

Calcium hydroxyapatite is derived from bone (bovine source) and therefore provides the optimum form of calcium for absorption into bones.

Most good calcium supplements will also include vitamin D3, and possibly boron, to help optimise absorption. Some may contain magnesium, due to the synergistic relationship

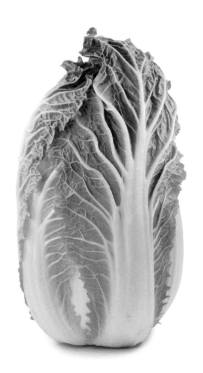

When should I take my supplement?

Calcium is best absorbed in doses of 500mg of elemental calcium or less. To optimise absorption, supplements are best consumed in smaller divided doses over the day rather than one large dose. Calcium is also well absorbed when the body is resting, therefore taking a dose at night is recommended.

Calcium citrate can be taken on an empty stomach whereas calcium carbonate should be consumed with food. All supplementary calcium should be taken away from your morning coffee.

What happens if I take too much?

Calcium is a very safe mineral with very low toxicity. The main side effect of excess consumption relates to the ingestion of excessive calcium carbonate, which can reduce stomach acid and lead to symptoms such as bloating, constipation, digestive discomfort.

Hypercalemia is a condition of too much calcium in the blood. This is rare and generally caused by a secondary disease or metabolic disorder.

between calcium and magnesium, however because these nutrients can compete for absorption they should ideally be taken away from each other, particularly for the elderly and those with poor digestion.

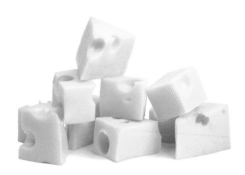

Matching it up

TAKE CALCIUM WITH

• Vitamin D

DON'T TAKE CALCIUM WITH

• Magnesium. Although these nutrients work together for muscle and bone health, they can compete for absorption during digestion and therefore should ideally be taken away from each other
• Caffeine can hinder absorption

Iodine

The Snapshot

Iodine is widely known for its antiseptic and antibacterial properties. Iodine tincture is a staple in most people's medicine cabinet, being used to treat minor cuts and abrasions. It's also a trace mineral and is essential to human life, vital for proper thyroid function and important during pregnancy for healthy brain development.

Other names

Potassium iodide or kelp is high in natural iodine.

What does it do?

Iodine is vital for the synthesis of the thyroid hormones thyroxine (T4) and triiodothyronine (T3). Thyroid hormones are responsible for the regulation of our metabolism and as such have an impact on every cell and virtually every physiological function in our body.

Iodine is essential for normal mental development of the foetus during pregnancy and maintenance of thyroid function. Iodine deficiency during pregnancy is the most common cause of preventable intellectual impairment worldwide and can lead to cretinism and failure to thrive in the infant. Adequate iodine may also play a role in the prevention of miscarriage.

Iodine is concentrated in breast milk for the benefit of the infant. A deficiency of iodine has been associated with changes in the breast tissue, known as atypia or dysplasia. These changes increase the risk of malignant tumour development. Treatment with therapeutic iodine has been shown to reverse these initial changes in some cases.

What foods does it come in?

Iodised salt	Fish	Cow's milk	Mozzarella cheese
Kelp and other	Shellfish	Eggs	Erythrosine (red
sea vegetables	Yoghurt	Strawberries	food colouring)

How do I know if I'm deficient?

Signs and Symtoms

MILD DEFICIENCY
- Impacts thyroid function and can cause enlargement and goiter formation

SEVERE DEFICIENCY
- Hypothyroidism

Is a supplement recommended for me?

Supplementation is recommended to maintain adequate iodine status during pregnancy. Supplements may also be beneficial to assist in the treatment of hypothyroidism but this should be monitored by a healthcare professional.

Matching it up

TAKE IODINE WITH
- Selenium to support thyroid hormone regulation

DON'T TAKE IODINE WITH
- Hyperthyroidism

Which supplement should I choose?

Iodine is commonly supplemented in the form of kelp supplements, which provide good doses of natural iodine, or in the form of potassium iodide. Potassium iodide is recommended during pregnancy whereas kelp can be useful for thyroid treatment.

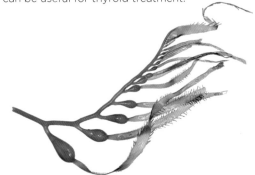

When should I take my supplement?

Kelp supplements should be taken with meals.

What happens if I take too much?

Acute toxicity of iodine is generally caused by ingestion of pure iodine, rather than the iodide form found in iodine supplements. This can be accidentally consumed in the form of antiseptic tincture and can produce toxic effects such as burning of the mouth, throat and stomach, stomach ache, diarrhoea and vomiting. In extreme cases it can lead to a weak pulse and coma.

How much should I have?

	AI	UL
INFANTS		
0 - 6 months	90mcg/day	Not possible to establish
7 - 12 months	110mcg/day	Not possible to establish
	RDI	**UL**
TODDLERS		
1 - 3 years	90mcg/day	200mcg/day
4 - 8 years	90mcg/day	300mcg/day
	RDI	**UL**
CHILDREN		
Boys 9 - 13 years	120mcg/day	600mcg/day
Boys 14 - 18 years	120mcg/day	900mcg/day
Girls 9 - 13 years	120mcg/day	600mcg/day
Girls 14 - 18 years	150mcg/day	900mcg/day
	RDI	**UL**
ADULTS		
Men 19 - 70 + years	150mcg/day	1100mcg/day
Women 19 - 70 + years	150mcg/day	1100mcg/day
	RDI	**UL**
PREGNANCY		
14 - 18 years	220mcg/day	900mcg/day
18 - 50 years	220mcg/day	1100mcg/day
	RDI	**UL**
LACTATION		
14 years	270mcg/day	900mcg/day
18 - 50 years	270mcg/day	1100mcg/day

It's very difficult to overdose on iodine through dietary sources or supplements containing iodine in the form of iodide. Even high intakes in this form are generally well tolerated, with Japanese people consuming as much as 12,000mcg daily through dietary sources alone. However, in susceptible individuals, high iodide intake can interfere with thyroid hormone production. In some cases it can actually mimic the symptoms of iodine deficiency. In other cases it can cause hyperthyroidism.

THERAPEUTIC ADULT DOSE

A supplement containing **220mg - 250mg** of iodine per day is recommended during pregnancy and breastfeeding. Other therapeutic supplementation should only be taken under the direction of a health care professional.

Iron

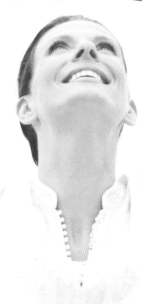

The Snapshot

Iron is essential to human life. It plays a major role in the transport of oxygen and carbon dioxide around the body as well as aiding the production of energy. It's required for synthesis of cellular DNA and also supports healthy immune function.

Demand for iron increases during all phases of rapid development including during pregnancy, infancy and teenage years. Supplemental iron can be beneficial during these times. However, iron is a heavy metal and is not easily excreted from the body, therefore supplementation should never exceed the recommended dose unless under the supervision of a health care professional.

Iron supplements are best consumed with vitamin C, in the form of iron amino acid chelate or ferros fumarate to optimise absorption and avoid constipation and gastric upset. Vitamin B12, B6 and folate are also important cofactors, alongside iron, in the maintenance of healthy red blood cells.

Other names

Ferros sulfate, ferros fumarate, iron amino acid chelate

What does it do?

Oxygen is required for the production and survival of all cells in the body and iron is essential to facilitate its transport, helping carry oxygen from the lungs to cells throughout the body and transport carbon dioxide back to our lungs for excretion. Around two thirds of our iron stores are found in haemoglobin, which is the protein in red blood cells that carries the oxygen for transport. Iron is also stored in myoglobin, which is a protein that helps transport oxygen to muscles; the remainder circulates through the body in blood plasma.

Iron also aids energy production by transporting oxygen to the mitochondria, which is the 'power house' of every cell, where energy is made.

DNA, which is the genetic 'blue print' upon which all our cells are built, requires iron for development. Iron is also required for protein metabolism, which further supports growth and development.

Immune cells require oxygen to facilitate oxygen dependent reactions, which allow them to kill invading bacteria and other pathogens. Iron is required to transport this oxygen to the immune cells.

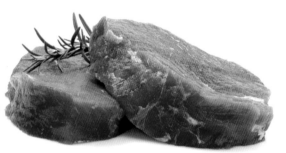

How do I know if I'm deficient?

Signs and Symtoms

MILD DEFICIENCY
- Weakness/fatigue
- Pallor
- Lack of concentration
- Dizziness
- Impaired immune function

SEVERE DEFICIENCY
- Anaemia
- Pregnant women with iron deficiency are more prone to spontaneous abortion, preterm delivery, stillbirth, low birth weight babies and post-delivery infection

What foods does it come in?

HEME IRON	Chicken	NON HEME IRON	Molasses
Liver	Pork	Soybeans	Spinach
Oysters	Tuna	Lentils	Tofu
Beef	Fish	Kidney beans	
Turkey			

Iron is better absorbed from meat (heme) sources than vegetarian (non-heme) sources.

Is a supplement recommended for me?

Demand for iron increases during all phases of rapid development including pregnancy, breastfeeding, infancy and the teenage years and supplemental iron can be beneficial during these times when increased demand for iron may not be met by dietary sources alone. Women with heavy menstrual bleeding may benefit from supplementation, as may those with gastrointestinal disorders affecting iron uptake. Preterm infants as well as older infants and toddlers may require supplementation during this growth phase if breast milk or dietary sources aren't sufficient to address demand. Those with iron deficiency anaemia are also recommended to consume iron supplements to improve iron stores.

How much should I have?

INFANTS	AI	UL
0 - 6 months	0.2mg/day	20mg/day
7 - 12 months	11mg/day	20mg/day
TODDLERS	**RDI**	**UL**
1 - 3 years	9mg/day	20mg/day
4 - 8 years	10mg/day	40mg/day
CHILDREN	**RDI**	**UL**
Boys 9 - 13 years	8mg/day	40mg/day
Boys 14 - 18 years	11mg/day	45mg/day
Girls 9 - 13 years	8mg/day	40mg/day
Girls 14 - 18 years	15mg/day	45mg/day
ADULTS	**RDI**	**UL**
Men 19 - 70 +years	8mg/day	45mg/day
Women 19 - 50 years	18mg/day	45mg/day
Women 50 - 70 + years	8mg/day	45mg/day
PREGNANCY	**RDI**	**UL**
14 + years	27mg/day	45mg/day
LACTATION	**RDI**	**UL**
14 - 18 years	10mg/day	45mg/day
18 - 50 years	9mg/day	45mg/day

THERAPEUTIC ADULT DOSE

Taking the RDI of iron is generally sufficient to provide therapeutic benefit.

Doses above the UL can be recommended for the treatment of iron deficiency anaemia. This is best taken in divided doses to avoid digestive upset and improve absorption and should only be taken under the direction of a health care professional.

Which supplement should I choose?

The most common supplemental sources of iron include ferros sulfate, ferros fumarate and iron amino acid chelate. Ferros sulfate has the poorest absorption, with around 20% being available for uptake. This form also commonly causes gut irritation and constipation. Ferros fumarate is a more natural source of Iron, with around 30% being available for absorption. Ferros fumarate is also less irritating to the gut and therefore less likely to cause side effects. Iron is best absorbed when in a chelated form, iron amino acid chelate, which means it is bound to other amino acids to enhance absorption. This form is also gentle on the stomach and the least likely to cause side effects. Natural liquid iron preparations can be beneficial to help optimise absorption for those with digestive difficulties.

When should I take my supplement?

Iron is ideally taken on an empty stomach away from food, tea, coffee and other caffeine containing beverages. However this may cause stomach upset in sensitive individuals and in this case supplements can be taken with a small amount of food. Ferros fumarate or sulfate supplements should also be consumed away from calcium, magnesium and zinc supplements. Iron supplements in a chelated form are less likely to interact with other minerals, so simultaneous consumption is less likely to pose problems.

Matching it up

TAKE IRON WITH
- Vitamin C to enhance absorption
- Folate, B6 and B12 work synergistically with iron to support healthy red blood cells

DON'T TAKE IRON WITH
- Calcium, magnesium, manganese, copper and zinc can compete for absorption

What happens if I take too much?

As iron is so essential to human life, to help ensure levels never become depleted, our body actually has no means by which to excrete iron. However, as a heavy metal, iron can also be potentially toxic; therefore uptake is tightly regulated by the body. If iron stores are high, the body actively decreases the amount of iron absorbed across through the gut. Therefore toxicity via dietary consumption is unlikely. However this absorption process can't be shut off entirely and stores can build up if excess supplemental iron is consumed. Excessive amounts of iron in circulation can cause critical damage to vital cells in the liver, heart and other vital organs, so high dose supplementation is not recommended unless under medical supervision.

Hemochromatosis is an inherited condition affecting the body's ability to regulate iron absorption. This leads to excess iron being absorbed and stored. This iron is stored in the liver, heart, pancreas, skin and other organs, generating free radicals which can seriously damage cells. The initial symptoms are generally fatigue, lethargy and achy joints. If left untreated, iron accumulation can lead to further complications including cancer, heart disease, arthritis, diabetes and liver disease. Early detection is vital to prevent potentially fatal outcomes; however this condition can often go undiagnosed until iron stores have reached 10-50 times the normal amount. Therefore early testing is advisable for those with a family history of the condition.

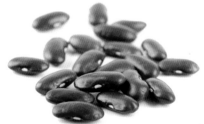

Magnesium

The Snapshot

Magnesium is another essential mineral involved in the basic structure of our DNA. Magnesium is a catalyst to over 300 enzymatic reactions in the body, with almost all our body systems relying on magnesium for their metabolic function.

Magnesium is known as a 'macromineral', which basically means we need lots of it. The body requires large amounts of magnesium to be delivered through the diet every day.

Muscle fatigue, cramps and spasms are the most common signs of deficiency and supplements are best taken in the form of a magnesium amino acid chelate, magnesium aspartate or magnesium orotate, or a combination of these, alongside vitamin B6 to enhance uptake.

Other names

Magnesium is not known by any other name.

What does it do?

Around two thirds of all magnesium in our body is stored in our bones. Some of this bone magnesium works in combination with calcium and phosphorus in the maintenance of the physical structure and strength of our bones. The remaining magnesium is stored on the outside surface of our bones. This surface magnesium doesn't appear to play a biologically active role but acts as a magnesium reserve from which the blood can draw upon as needed, if dietary supply is inadequate.

Magnesium works in combination with calcium in the regulation of the nervous and musculoskeletal system, to make sure they're communicating effectively with each other. Calcium is required to activate nerve cells, which send signals to stimulate the muscles. Magnesium helps to regulate these signals and block any excess activation, which can cause excess muscle stimulation and cramping. Via this process, magnesium helps maintain muscles in a relaxed state, preventing cramps, twitches and tension.

As the heart is a large muscle, magnesium works in a similar manner on the heart muscle to support the regulation of normal heart rhythm and blood pressure. Magnesium also plays an important role in carbohydrate metabolism and is involved in the release of insulin.

How do I know if I'm deficient?

Due to the involvement of magnesium in a wide variety of body systems, deficiency can have a widespread impact on the body and deficiency symptoms can vary greatly. The main symptoms of deficiency affect the muscles, including cramps, spasms and fatigue. Those with poorly controlled diabetes are at greater risk of deficiency. This is due to the fact that their requirements can be higher because of the involvement of magnesium in blood sugar regulation as well as the fact that their urinary excretion can be higher, as occurs during episodes of hyperglycemia.

Signs and Symtoms

MILD DEFICIENCY

- Muscle fatigue
- Muscle cramps and spasms
- Restless leg syndrome
- Low mood/depression
- Poor blood sugar regulation
- Headaches

SEVERE DEFICIENCY

- Arrhythmia
- Irregular heart beat
- Increased heart rate
- Increased blood pressure
- Lack of appetite
- Bone fractures and osteoporosis

What foods does it come in?

Pumpkin seeds	Halibut	Lentils	Raisins
Spinach and other green vegetables	Black beans	Oats	Milk
	Kidney beans	Wheat germ	Chocolate
Soybeans	Almonds	Unrefined whole grains	
Sunflower seeds	Cashews		
Sesame seeds	Peanuts	Bananas	

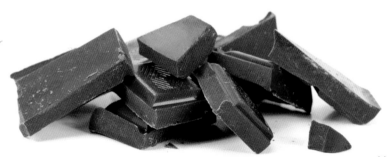

How much should I have?

	AI	UL (as a supplement)
INFANTS		
0 – 6 months	30mg/day	Not possible to establish
7 – 12 months	75mg/day	Not possible to establish

	RDI	UL (as a supplement)
TODDLERS		
1 – 3 years	80mg/day	65mg/day
4 – 8 years	130mg/day	110mg/day

	RDI	UL (as a supplement)
CHILDREN		
Boys 9 – 13 years	240mg/day	350mg/day
Boys 14 – 18 years	410mg/day	350mg/day
Girls 9 – 13 years	240mg/day	350mg/day
Girls 14 – 18 years	360mg/day	350mg/day

	RDI	UL (as a supplement)
ADULTS		
Men 19 – 30 years	400mg/day	350mg/day
Men 30 – 70 + years	420mg/day	350mg/day
Women 19 – 30 years	310mg/day	350mg/day
Women 30 – 70 + years	320mg/day	350mg/day

	RDI	UL (as a supplement)
PREGNANCY		
14 – 18 years	400mg/day	350mg/day
19 – 30 years	350mg/day	350mg/day
30 – 50 years	360mg/day	350mg/day

	RDI	UL (as a supplement)
LACTATION		
14 – 18 years	360mg/day	350mg/day
19 – 30 years	310mg/day	350mg/day
30 – 50 years	320mg/day	350mg/day

THERAPEUTIC ADULT DOSE

100-250mg of elemental magnesium per day is a good supplemental maintenance dose in the regulation of blood pressure, arrhythmia, blood sugar control and prevention of cramps and spasms. **250mg - 350mg** is recommended as a therapeutic dose in the treatment of the above conditions. Due to its involvement in the regulation of heart rhythm, magnesium is often given intravenously in higher doses in the treatment of arrhythmia.

Is a supplement recommended for me?

Those suffering from muscular cramps and spasms, tension, twitches or restless leg syndrome can benefit from magnesium supplements to help prevent and relieve these symptoms. Athletes or those participating in strenuous exercise can also benefit from magnesium supplementation to help prevent muscular cramps during and after exercise. The elderly are at greater risk of deficiency due to decreased uptake and metabolism therefore supplementation can be useful in these later years.

Diuretics can increase the amount of magnesium lost through urine therefore supplementation may be beneficial for these individuals, as well as those with poorly controlled diabetes. However a health care professional should be consulted in these conditions.

Which supplement should I choose?

Magnesium oxide is one of the cheapest and most common sources of magnesium. Magnesium oxide provides the largest amount of magnesium and will significantly boost the magnesium content in supplements; however this source also provides the lowest rate of absorption. Magnesium oxide is commonly used as a laxative and therefore can also cause diarrhoea and gastric upset.

Magnesium citrate, aspartate, orotate and amino acid chelate provide better absorption and are therefore the best forms to look for in a supplement. Ideally a combination of these forms, as magnesium is better absorbed when provided in a variety of forms rather than a higher dose of one. Vitamin B6 is also required for optimal transfer of magnesium into cells therefore a supplement which also contains vitamin B6 is optimal.

When should I take my supplement?

To optimise absorption magnesium is best taken between meals away from food. As a natural relaxant, magnesium is good to take at night before bed to help promote relaxation and sleep. If taking higher therapeutic doses, these are best spread out over the day.

What happens if I take too much?

Excess magnesium in the blood is easily filtered and excreted through the kidneys therefore it is difficult to overdose on magnesium through dietary sources. The main toxicity symptom experienced from excessive supplementation is diarrhoea and abdominal cramping. This is particularly common if taking magnesium oxide. Excess long term magnesium build up can cause symptoms including nausea, loss of appetite, muscle weakness, altered mental state, breathing difficulties, severely low blood pressure and irregular heartbeat.

Matching it up

TAKE MAGNESIUM WITH
- Potassium
- Vitamin B6

DON'T TAKE MAGNESIUM WITH
- Calcium and magnesium can compete for absorption

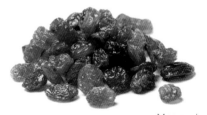

Selenium

The Snapshot

Selenium is a powerful antioxidant and is also involved in healthy thyroid function. Supplementation can be beneficial to improve antioxidant capacity, helping to reduce signs of aging, aid in the prevention of some cancers and improve fertility. The antioxidant capacity of selenium is strongest when supplemented with vitamin E.

Other names

Selenium is not known by any other name.

What does it do?

Selenium is another one of our 'bodyguard' nutrients, acting as a powerful antioxidant, preventing cells from oxidative damage due to aging and environmental exposure. Selenium is an important cofactor to one of the body's most important antioxidant and detoxification enzymes, glutathione peroxidase. It can assist in the prevention of subsequent conditions relating to oxidative stress including cardiovascular disease, rheumatoid arthritis, infertility, chronic fatigue and it can assist in slowing the aging process.

As a potent antioxidant, selenium has been particularly implicated in cancer prevention. Various mechanisms for this anti cancer activity have been suggested including its potential role in the repair of damaged cells, inhibition of proliferation of cancer cells and increased elimination of damaged cells.

Selenium works in combination with iodine to maintain healthy thyroid function and is essential in the regulation of thyroid hormones.

How do I know if I'm deficient?

Symptoms of true selenium deficiency are hard to determine and mild deficiency doesn't appear to produce any noticeable symptoms.

Signs and Symtoms

MILD DEFICIENCY
- None known

SEVERE DEFICIENCY
- Impaired thyroid function
- Joint pain or weakness

What foods does it come in?

Brazil nuts (highest known dietary source of selenium)	Kidney Crab Tuna	Lobster Meat Corn	Wheat Soybean

Is a supplement recommended for me?

Due to its antioxidant capacity, selenium may be beneficial in the treatment and prevention of cancer; however with the conflicting evidence for use in prostate cancer, it should only be used under advisement of your health care professional in this case. Supplementation can be beneficial to support fertility in both males and females, however excess intake may affect sperm motility so dosing should not exceed therapeutic recommendations.

Matching it up

TAKE SELENIUM WITH
- Vitamin E

DON'T TAKE SELENIUM WITH
- Caution when prostate cancer is present

Which supplement should I choose?

Supplements are generally available in the form of selenomethionine, sodium selenite and sodium selenate. Some supplements may also contain selenium in a yeast form. Both sodium selenite and sodium selenate are inorganic forms of selenium therefore selenomethionine is recommended as the best absorbed and utilised form.

When should I take my supplement?

There is little evidence to suggest whether selenium is better taken with or without food. If the supplement also contains vitamin E it is recommended to take with food.

How much should I have?

	AI	UL
INFANTS		
0 – 6 months	12mcg/day	45mcg/day
7 – 12 months	15mcg/day	60mcg/day
TODDLERS	RDI	UL
1 – 3 years	25mcg/day	90mcg/day
4 – 8 years	30mcg/day	150mcg/day
CHILDREN	RDI	UL
Boys 9 – 13 years	50mcg/day	280mcg/day
Boys 14 – 18 years	70mcg/day	400mcg/day
Girls 9 – 13 years	50mcg/day	280mcg/day
Girls 14 – 18 years	60mcg/day	400mcg/day
ADULTS	RDI	UL
Men 19 – 70 + years	70mcg/day	400mcg/day
Women 19 – 70 + years	60mcg/day	400mcg/day
PREGNANCY	RDI	UL
14 + years	65mcg/day	400mcg/day
LACTATION	RDI	UL
14 + years	75mcg/day	400mcg/day

THERAPEUTIC ADULT DOSE

50mcg - 160mcg is the optimal treatment dose for maximum antioxidant activity. Higher doses may be prescribed for by health care professionals for thyroid and cancer treatment.

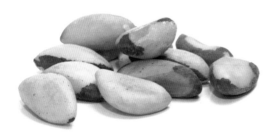

What happens if I take too much?

Selenium is toxic in high doses leading to a condition known as selenosis. Symptoms include gastrointestinal disturbance, halitosis (particularly a garlic-like odour on the breath), hair loss, flaking nails, fatigue, irritability and neurological damage. If left untreated selenosis can cause pulmonary odema and cirrhosis of the liver and can be fatal. For this reason it is recommended that a daily dietary intake of 400mcg not be exceeded.

Zinc

The Snapshot

Zinc is an essential trace element, vital to the survival of humans, animals, plants and all microorganisms. Zinc is involved in maintaining a healthy immune system, good digestion and metabolism as well as being involved in our taste and smell receptors. Hormones in both males and females require adequate zinc for healthy regulation and it's particularly important during times of growth, development and repair including conception and pregnancy.

Other names

Zinc is not known by any other name.

What does it do?

Zinc is involved in the breakdown and utilisation of carbohydrates, fat and proteins in the digestive system. It's also required for the activation, synthesis and utilisation of insulin and helps protect the beta cells, which produce insulin, against damage. Insulin is required to regulate blood sugar levels.

Zinc is essential for optimal functioning of the immune system. It helps support thymus gland function and assists in the production of our body's 'infection fighting army', the white blood cells.

Zinc helps promote healthy functioning of the major organs of the hormonal system, the thyroid, the pituitary, the adrenal glands, the ovaries and the testes, and plays a role in the metabolism of oestrogen and testosterone. Zinc is important in males for healthy functioning of the prostate and regulation of testosterone and supports ovulation in females. Zinc helps regulate the conversion of testosterone into its more active form and helps control the uptake of testosterone by the prostate. With its key role in hormone production and balance, zinc is essential for fertility in females and males.

Zinc is also involved in growth and repair of tissue, for the synthesis of DNA, division and replication of cells as well as the structure and function of our cell walls. For this reason it is essential for healthy growth and development of the foetus during pregnancy and via its role in tissue regeneration, it can also help prevent associated stretch marks!

Zinc is required to support the health of the skin via its role in wound healing, inflammation control and tissue regeneration. It is also important in the regulation of the skin's oil balance and for the production of collagen, which is essential for strength and growth of bones, nails and hair.

Zinc is utilised in the brain for the production of neurotransmitters, which transport messages from the brain to our muscles. Zinc is the most abundant trace mineral in the eye. It's required for maintenance of healthy vision and has been shown to play a role in the prevention of macular degeneration.

Zinc is required for the production of hydrochloric acid in the stomach, which is essential for healthy digestion. It's also important for the healthy functioning of our taste and smell receptors. This is one of the reasons why you can lose your sense of taste when you've got a cold, because all your zinc is being used to fight the infection.

How do I know if I'm deficient?

As zinc plays such a major role in the function of many of our major organs and systems, symptoms of zinc deficiency can be widespread and deficiency is relatively common. Women taking the pill can be at greater risk of deficiency as it can reduce zinc levels. Vegetarians are also at increased risk as zinc is better absorbed from animal sources. Phytic acid, found in fibrous fruits, vegetables and whole grains can impair absorption.

Zinc deficiency is often tested by way of a taste test. Due to the involvement of zinc in our taste and smell receptors, a decreased ability to taste a specially prepared zinc solution (available over the counter in pharmacies or health food stores) can indicate low zinc levels.

Signs and Symtoms

MILD DEFICIENCY

- Hair loss
- Brittle nails
- White spots on nails
- Impaired immune function and healing capacity
- Impaired growth and development
- Decreased fertility in men and women

SEVERE DEFICIENCY

- Can cause birth defects, low birth weight, spontaneous abortion, premature delivery, impaired brain development, mental retardation and behavioural problems in the infant during pregnancy.

What foods does it come in?

Liver	Canned fish	Chicken	Nuts
Oysters	Red meat	Eggs	Pulses
Shellfish	Pork	Hard cheese	Whole grains

Is a supplement recommended for me?

Zinc can be beneficial to help reduce the severity and duration of cold and flu symptoms and speed recovery from infection. It can also support recovery from injury and surgery by supporting healing. Supplementation can also be used to treat skin conditions such as acne and eczema. Supplementation can be particularly beneficial in hormonal acne due to its action on the hormonal system, skin sebum balance and skin repair.

Supplements can be useful preconception to support fertility in both males and females. Supplementation can be particularly beneficial for women who have previously taken the pill, as this can deplete zinc stores. Supplementation during pregnancy has been shown to aid healthy growth and improve birth weight, as well as helping to reduce incidence of cold/flu and infection in the mother.

Zinc supplementation has been used in the treatment of anorexia nervosa, as those suffering this condition are often found to be deficient. Supplementation can aid in recovery by stimulating taste and smell receptors, improving perception of taste.

Benign prostatic hyperplasia or enlarged prostate can benefit from zinc supplementation to help reduce enlargement and alleviate symptoms. This therapeutic effect is thought to be due to its multi-factorial effect on the hormonal system in reducing excess conversion of testosterone into its active form, inhibiting the binding of hormones to receptor cells and helping to lower the uptake of testosterone by the prostate which helps reduce prostate growth.

Zinc supplements are proving to be effective in reducing the progression of macular degeneration, particularly when combined with other antioxidant nutrients.

Phytic acid or phytate, commonly found in the fibre portion of fruits, vegetables and whole grains can bind to zinc and decrease absorption. This means that approximately 15% of zinc is absorbed from a high phytate diet compared to around 40% from a diet high in animal protein. Vegetarian diets, which are naturally high in phytic acid, can lead to a decreased absorption of zinc. Zinc is also better absorbed through protein sources, so those following a vegetarian diet may have an increased requirement for zinc and supplementation may be beneficial.

Which supplement should I choose?

Zinc supplements are generally available in the form of zinc sulfate or zinc oxide, which are inorganic forms, or as an amino acid chelate, which means it is bound to another molecule. Zinc needs to bind with other molecules for absorption in the diet so a chelated zinc is the best supplemental source to look for.

Zinc chelates fall into two common categories, those bound to organic acids and those bound to amino acids. The organic acids commonly used include picolinic acid, orotic acid, citric acid and gluconic acid. The amino acids used commonly include methionine, monomethionine and aspartic acid. Supplement labels may list the nutrient as zinc amino acid chelate, or it may list the molecule to which it's bound e.g. zinc gluconate, zinc picolinate, zinc citrate, zinc aspartate etc. All provide varying amounts of elemental zinc however there is little evidence suggesting benefits of one chelated source over another.

Lozenge forms are also available and can be beneficial in acute treatment of coughs and sore throat.

How much should I have?

	AI	UL
INFANTS		
0 – 6 months	2mg/day	4mg/day
7 – 12 months	3mg/day	5mg/day

	RDI	UL
TODDLERS		
1 – 3 years	3mg/day	7mg/day
4 – 8 years	4mg/day	12mg/day

	RDI	UL
CHILDREN		
Boys 9 – 13 years	6mg/day	25mg/day
Boys 14 – 18 years	13mg/day	34mg/day
Girls 9 – 13 years	6mg/day	25mg/day
Girls 14 – 18 years	7mg/day	35mg/day

	RDI	UL
ADULTS		
Men 19 – 70 + years	14mg/day	40mg/day
Women 19 – 70 + years	8mg/day	40mg/day

	RDI	UL
PREGNANCY		
14 – 18 years	10mg/day	35mg/day
19 – 50 years	11mg/day	40mg/day

	RDI	UL
LACTATION		
14 – 18 years	9mg/day	35mg/day
19 + years	10mg/day	40mg/day

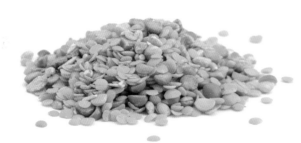

THERAPEUTIC ADULT DOSE

12 - 24mg is a good therapeutic dose to boost the immune system during infection, promote healing, assist in the treatment of acne and assist in the treatment and prevention of macular degeneration.

The RDI is generally sufficient to support fertility, insulin regulation, metabolism, digestion and brain and eye health.

Zinc and copper function synergistically in many of their metabolic functions so the body requires a balanced amount of both nutrients. Excessive intake of zinc can lead to a deficiency of copper; conversely excess copper can reduce zinc levels. Zinc may also be used to intentionally reduce copper levels where excess exists.

When should I take my supplement?

Absorption of zinc can be impaired by simultaneous consumption of phytic acid, found in the fibre portion of fruits, vegetables and whole grains, therefore zinc supplements are generally better absorbed when taken away from these foods. Zinc supplements are absorbed well on an empty stomach; however this may cause nausea in sensitive individuals and should be taken after meals if this occurs.

What happens if I take too much?

Excess intake of zinc can be harmful, although toxicity via oral ingestion is rare as the body will generally induce a vomit reflex if high doses are consumed. Taking prolonged high doses (over 50mg per day) may cause a secondary deficiency of copper and excessive doses (as with deficiency) may interfere with the sense of smell, while headaches and dizziness have also been noted. Doses above 150mg may have a reverse effect on the immune system by impairing immune function. Zinc oxide and zinc chloride, used for industrial purposes, can be toxic if excess is inhaled.

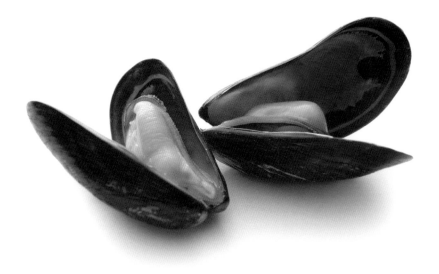

Other Important Nutrients

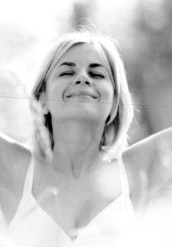

Coenzyme Q10

The Snapshot

Coenzyme Q10 is found in all living cells and is vital for the production of energy. It is essential for heart heath and possesses potent antioxidant activity. Our body can naturally produce coenzyme Q10, therefore there is no recognised RDI or AI, however supplementation can be beneficial to improve energy, help reduce the signs of aging and improve heart health. Statin cholesterol medications reduce the body's ability to produce coenzyme Q10; leading to side effects such as muscle aches and fatigue, therefore supplements can be beneficial with these medications.

Other names

CoQ10

What does it do?

Coenzyme Q10 is a naturally occurring nutrient, which is present in all cells. It is most concentrated in the mitochondria, which is where energy is produced, as it is vital for energy production.

The heart contains the highest concentration of coenzyme Q10 as it has the highest demand for cellular energy. Coenzyme Q10 is an essential nutrient for heart health due to its ability to provide vital energy for heart function as well as helping to inhibit blood clot formation and provide potent antioxidant activity. Coenzyme Q10 has also been shown to assist in the reduction of high blood pressure as well as helping to reduce the oxidation of cholesterol, which can lead to atherosclerosis.

Coenzyme Q10 is an excellent cellular 'bodyguard' nutrient, possessing potent antioxidant properties to help protect our cells from oxidative damage caused by environmental exposure and aging. As we age, our body's natural production of coenzyme Q10 gradually decreases, so supplementation becomes more important the older we get.

How do I know if I'm deficient?

Signs and Symtoms

MILD DEFICIENCY
- Lack of energy
- Muscle aches and fatigue

SEVERE DEFICIENCY
- Rare, generally caused by medications disrupting natural production such as statin cholesterol medications. Can cause severe muscle aches and fatigue and increase the risk of cardiovascular disease

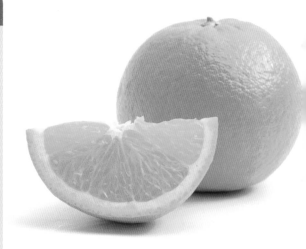

Co Enzyme Q10 is available in a variety of foods but meat and fish are the richest sources.

What foods does it come in?

Beef	White fish	Walnuts	Grapes
Heart	Salmon	Sesame seeds	Avocado
Liver	Tuna	Pistachio nuts	Blackcurrants
Pork	Soy bean oil	Hazelnuts	Strawberries
Chicken	Olive oil	Almonds	Oranges
Sardines	Grapeseed oil	Broccoli	
Mackerel	Sunflower oil	Parsley	
Red fish	Peanuts	Cauliflower	

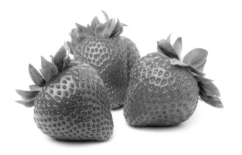

How much should I have?

THERAPEUTIC ADULT DOSE

100 - 300mg is the recommended dose for therapeutic benefit.
50 - 150mg is sufficient to maintain general health.

Is a supplement recommended for me?

Coenzyme Q10 is a vital nutrient for heart health and supplementation can be beneficial for those with cardiovascular issues including high blood pressure and arrhythmia or those with a family history of cardiovascular disease. Those taking statin medications to reduce cholesterol will benefit from supplementation as statin medications reduce the body's ability to produce coenzyme Q10, resulting in the common side effect of muscle aches/fatigue.

As an antioxidant nutrient, coenzyme Q10 is contained in many beauty creams and can be beneficial as a supplement to help reduce the signs of aging.

Which supplement should I choose?

Coenzyme Q10 is best absorbed in a capsule or soft gel form rather than tablet.

Matching it up

TAKE COENZYME Q10 WITH
- Beneficial when taken with magnesium to support healthy blood pressure
- Beneficial when taken with the B vitamins to support energy production

DON'T TAKE COENZYME Q10 WITH
- Caution when taking with warfarin

When should I take my supplement?

Coenzyme Q10 is best taken with food.

What happens if I take too much?

Coenzyme Q10 has not been shown to have any toxicity.

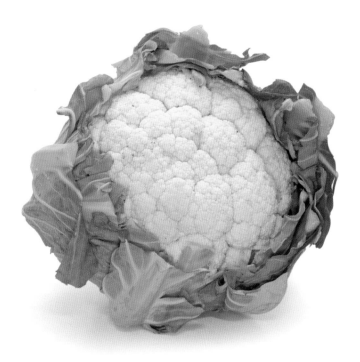

Lysine

The Snapshot

As with all amino acids, lysine is an essential building block for protein, assisting in muscle growth and development and the absorption of calcium for bone health. However the most well known role of lysine is in the treatment and prevention of cold sores.

Other names

Lysine is not known by any other name.

What does it do?

Lysine is widely recognised for its role in the treatment and prevention of cold sores by competing with and blocking the effect of arginine. About 90% of the world's population carry the herpes simplex virus, which creates cold sores. The majority of the time this virus lays dormant in nerve roots and can be activated by low immunity and stress. Arginine is required to complete this activation and cause a cold sore lesion as well as other symptoms of the herpes virus.

Having sufficient levels of lysine in your system reduces your arginine stores. This helps to reduce the incidence and also reduce the duration and severity of a cold sore break out.

Lysine is an amino acid and as such is essential for muscle growth and development. Lysine can also support bone health by assisting the absorption of calcium.

How do I know if I'm deficient?

Signs and Symtoms

MILD DEFICIENCY

- Fatigue
- Nausea
- Loss of appetite
- Irritability
- Coldsore outbreaks

SEVERE DEFICIENCY

- Dizziness
- Bloodshot eyes
- Impaired growth
- Reproductive disorders

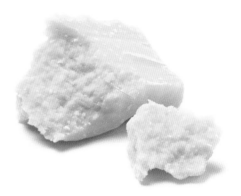

Chocolate and nuts are high in arginine, which can reduce lysine levels and spark cold sore production; these foods should be avoided in those suffering cold sores.

What foods does it come in?

Chicken	Lentils	Cheese (particularly	Aduki beans
Beef	Kidney beans	parmesan)	Milk
Lamb	Split peas	Fish (particularly	Eggs
Pork	Chickpeas	catfish, cod and	Nuts
Soybeans	Amaranth	sardines)	Brewer's yeast

How much should I have?

Lysine is not considered an essential nutrient and therefore no RDI or AI has been set.

THERAPEUTIC ADULT DOSE

For the treatment of cold sores it is recommended to take a dose of **1500mg – 4000mg** per day until the lesion subsides. This can be reduced to a dose of around **500 - 750mg** as a preventative measure.

Is a supplement recommended for me?

Lysine supplements can assist in the prevention and treatment of cold sore outbreaks and other symptoms associated with the herpes virus.

Which supplement should I choose?

Most supplements will contain between 500mg - 1000mg of lysine. To further aid in the treatment of cold sores it may also be beneficial to look for a supplement which contains other immune boosting nutrients such as zinc, vitamin A and vitamin C.

When should I take my supplement?

Lysine is best absorbed when taken on an empty stomach.

Matching it up

TAKE LYSINE WITH
- Can support calcium uptake
- Vitamin C, vitamin A and zinc for improved healing of cold sore outbreaks

DON'T TAKE LYSINE WITH
- Arginine can compete for absorption

What happens if I take too much?

There have been no reports of toxicity with oral doses of lysine.

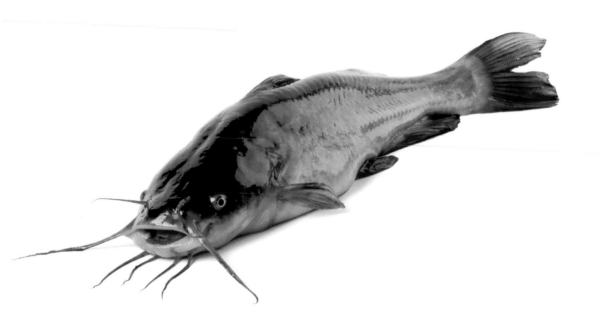

Omega 3

The Snapshot

Omega 3, mainly derived from fish oil and flaxseed oil, is part of the family of omega nutrients including omega 6 and 9, which fall under the banner of 'essential fatty acids'. They are classed as 'essential' as they are required for many functions within the body, yet we cannot manufacture them ourselves and instead adequate supply must be consumed through the diet. The active constituents of omega 3 fatty acids are EPA (eicosapentaenoic acid) and DHA (docosahexaenoic acid).

Omega 3 can help reduce inflammation, support cardiovascular and brain health, support foetal brain development during pregnancy and it has the extra benefit of helping to keep skin supple and reduce stretch marks. All cell membranes require omega 3 and an increased intake can help improve the condition of hair, skin and nails.

Other names

Linoleic acid

What does it do?

Omega 3, particularly the EPA component, possesses natural anti-inflammatory properties. It achieves this by reducing the production and effectiveness of the prostaglandins, which accelerate inflammation.

Omega 3, particularly the DHA content, has been shown to be beneficial in brain development and cognitive function, especially in infants, children and the elderly. During pregnancy and breastfeeding, omega 3 supports healthy brain development in the foetus as well as keeping mother's skin soft and supple, helping to reduce stretch marks. DHA has also been found to assist in the treatment and prevention of mood disorders including ADD and ADHD in children, as well as anxiety and depression. DHA again plays an important role in maintaining brain function in the elderly and may assist in the treatment and prevention of conditions such as Alzheimer's disease and dementia.

Omega 3 can be found in the lipid (fat) layer surrounding every cell in our body. This omega 3 content helps keep our cells supple. Increased omega

3 intake can help improve the appearance of dry/aging skin, can help improve dry/brittle nails and maintain hair strength and shine. With its additional anti-inflammatory action, omega 3 also assists in the treatment of eczema, psoriasis and dermatitis by helping to reduce redness and itching, and improving moisture.

There is strong evidence for the use of omega 3 in the prevention and treatment of cardiovascular disease. Increased intake of this essential fatty acid has been shown to help reduce cholesterol, assist in the reduction of blood pressure and arrhythmia, help prevent atherosclerosis and reduce the risk of heart attack. The EPA content of fish oil has been shown to be the most important constituent in relation to heart health.

How do I know if I'm deficient?

Signs and Symtoms

MILD DEFICIENCY
- Dry skin and brittle nails
- Exacerbation of inflammatory conditions

SEVERE DEFICIENCY
- May affect foetal brain development during pregnancy.

What foods does it come in?

Salmon	Scallops	Flaxseeds	Cauliflower
Sardines	Shrimp	Soybeans	Mustard seeds
Halibut	Cod	Tofu	Cabbage
Snapper	Red fish	Miso	Broccoli
Tuna	White fish	Walnuts	Brussels sprouts

How much should I have?

There is no established RDI for omega 3. Consumption of around 180 – 540mg of EPA and 120 - 360mg of DHA per day is beneficial to support brain and general health. This dose can be found in 1 - 3 standard 1000mg fish oil capsules.

THERAPEUTIC ADULT DOSE

At least 1800mg of EPA and 1200mg of DHA is recommended to reduce inflammation and provide cardiovascular benefit. This can be found in 6 - 12 standard Fish Oil capsules or 3 - 6 high strength capsules.

250mg – 2500mg of DHA is recommended to support foetal brain development during pregnancy, with doses above 1200mg per day showing benefits of increase cognitive function and IQ scores in children.

Is a supplement recommended for me?

Supplements can be beneficial to relieve the pain and inflammation of arthritis or other inflammatory conditions and assist in the treatment of eczema. Omega 3 and the active constituent DHA in particular, can be beneficial to support memory and brain function. Supplements are recommended during pregnancy and breastfeeding to ensure optimal brain development of the infant as well as helping to prevent stretch marks and post natal depression in the mother.

Which supplement should I choose?

When choosing an omega 3 supplement, fish oil is the best source as it is the most easily metabolised. Omega 3 is also available through flaxseed oil supplements, which contain omega 3, 6 and 9 and is a good option for vegetarians. However, metabolism of omega 3 from flaxseed oil requires an additional step in the metabolic process, which may hinder absorption in some people.

When choosing a fish oil supplement, the main thing to look for is the EPA and DHA content. These are the active constituents of omega 3, therefore the higher the EPA/DHA content the more potent the therapeutic benefit. Most standard 1000mg fish oil capsules will contain 180mg of EPA and 120mg of DHA, however high strength liquids and capsules can provide much higher doses of EPA and DHA, which will provide stronger therapeutic activity.

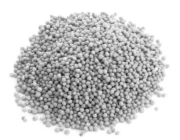

Omega 3 oils are particularly susceptible to damage from heat, light and oxygen. Therefore supplements should be bought and stored in airtight, dark glass or plastic containers and stored away from heat and light. If the supplement is in liquid form, not capsulated, this should be refrigerated after opening. A good quality supplement should not cause a 'fishy' aftertaste.

Matching it up

TAKE OMEGA 3 WITH

- Adequate vitamin B6, vitamin B3, vitamin C, magnesium and zinc are required for optimal omega 3 absorption

DON'T TAKE OMEGA 3 WITH

- Caution with warfarin or bleeding disorders as it can assist in thinning the blood

When should I take my supplement?

Omega 3 supplements are best taken with food.

What happens if I take too much?

Essential fatty acids are very safe with the only possible side effect of extreme excessive consumption being weight gain. Excess fatty acids which are not otherwise used by the body can be stored as fat. This is highly unlikely to occur through general supplementation unless doses far beyond therapeutic recommendations are consumed.

Probiotics

The Snapshot

The term probiotic originates from the Greek language and means 'for life', indicating the opposite of antibiotic. The current definition as accepted by the World Health Organization is "Live organisms when administered in adequate amounts confer a health benefit on the host". Most people generally recognise probiotics as the 'good bacteria' that colonise our digestive system.

The most commonly used probiotics fall into two categories, lactic acid bacteria (lactobacillus) or bifidobacteria. Lactobacillus is the most abundant strain in the adult digestive system whereas the infant and child's digestive system is dominated by bifidobacterium. This balance gradually begins to change at around seven years of age.

Probiotics also support the immune system to fight infection as well as helping to reduce eczema and allergy.

Other names

Probiotics are often referred to as acidophilus, however this is simply the most common strain of probiotic.

What does it do?

Bacteria in the colon plays a key role in the breakdown and metabolism of our food, the absorption of nutrients and the general maintenance of a healthy digestive system, assisting in the prevention of bloating, constipation, diarrhoea and heartburn, and in the treatment of irritable bowel syndrome (IBS).

Certain strains of probiotics, particularly lactobacillus plantarum, have shown beneficial effects in the treatment of inflammatory conditions such as inflammatory bowel disease (IBD).

Lactobacillius bacteria helps convert lactose into lactic acid. This can help improve the lactose metabolism and thus relieve the symptoms associated with lactose intolerance.

Seventy per cent of our immune function stems from our digestive system. A healthy digestive system with a balance of good bacteria ensures important nutrients from our food are being absorbed and that harmful substances are being excreted, helping to prevent infection and ensure optimum nutrition. A digestive environment with low levels of good bacteria is more susceptible to invasion of harmful pathogenic bacteria.

Probiotics are particularly beneficial for the treatment of fungal infections including thrush and candida, as they help prevent the colonisation of the fungi causing these infections. This reduces the severity and duration of symptoms and helps prevent further outbreaks. This immune activity can be beneficial during pregnancy to help protect against cold and flu as well as helping to protect against pregnancy complications and infection caused by pathogenic organisms. Probiotics can also aid the absorption of vital nutrients and help prevent common pregnancy symptoms such as heartburn and constipation by improving digestion.

Probiotic supplements can be of benefit in the treatment of childhood eczema and allergies. These conditions are caused by an 'overreaction' of the immune system, causing it to react to substances which should otherwise be innocuous. Probiotics can help rebalance the immune system and lessen the allergic reaction, assisting in the reduction of symptoms and in some cases preventing longer term allergy/eczema symptoms. Supplementation has shown to be of most benefit in children rather than adults, as once the immune system has developed there is less ability to reverse the allergic potential.

Antibiotics kill off "bad" invading bacteria to fight infection, however during this process they can also kill off our "good" beneficial bacteria. Probiotics can help recolonise the gut with healthy bacteria to rebalance the digestive system following antibiotic use.

How do I know if I'm deficient?

Signs and Symtoms

MILD DEFICIENCY

- Bloating
- Indigestion
- Constipation
- Diarrhoea
- Low resistance to infection, particularly candida and thrush
- Reduced nutrient absorption

SEVERE DEFICIENCY

- Malnutrition

The processing of these foods can destroy the live bacteria so they should be consumed in their natural state for maximum benefits.

What foods does it come in?

Yoghurt (naturally set is best)	Cottage cheese Buttermilk	Miso Tempeh	Kefir Sauerkraut

How much should I have?

There is no recognised RDI for probiotics, however most people can benefit from the introduction of around 10-50 billion live bacteria per day.

Is a supplement recommended for me?

Probiotic supplements can be beneficial to support the health of the digestive system in those experiencing bloating, constipation, diarrhoea, heartburn and general digestive difficulties as well as those with clinically diagnosed irritable bowel syndrome (IBS), inflammatory bowel disease (IBD) or lactose intolerance.

Probiotic supplements are recommended following antibiotic therapy to replace beneficial bacteria, which may have been killed off during the course of treatment. In this instance, the probiotic supplements should be taken during the course of antibiotics, at least one hour away from the antibiotic dose and for at least two weeks after the antibiotic course has been completed.

Children with eczema, asthma or other allergic conditions can benefit from the introduction of probiotic supplements.

THERAPEUTIC ADULT DOSE

10 - 20 billion live bacteria per day is beneficial in maintaining general health of the digestive system.
20 - 50 billion live bacteria per day is recommended if using therapeutically to treat specific symptoms.

Supplementation can also be beneficial in pregnancy to help improve digestion and relieve symptoms such as heartburn and constipation.

Which supplement should I choose?

As probiotics are live bacteria they should be kept refrigerated. Always ensure your supplement has been refrigerated when purchased. If left unrefrigerated, the bacteria will not 'go off' they will simply lose their potency. Some supplements claim to be room temperature stable but these should be treated with caution.

Most bacteria are not able to survive the high acid environment of the stomach to reach the intestines where they are most active, therefore it is ideal to look for a supplement which is labelled acid resistant or enteric coated.

There are also a variety of probiotic strains that have specific benefits for various conditions.

General Health and Digestion

As the most common strain in the adult digestive system, L. acidophilus is the strain most commonly available in supplements and is a good strain to look for to support general digestive health. However, as the balance of good bacteria is unique to each individual, some people may experience more benefit from a probiotic supplement containing a variety of bacterial strains.

Inflammation

When treating inflammatory conditions lactobacillus plantarum is the best strain to look for. This strain can also be beneficial in the treatment of some cases of irritable bowel syndrome where inflammation is present.

Children

When treating children under the age of seven years, the best strains to look for are bifidobacterium infantis, bifidobacterium breve and bifidobacterium longum as these are the most abundant strains in the developing digestive system.

Thrush/Candida

Those suffering from thrush can benefit from supplements as per the general recommendations; however one of the best strains for the treatment and prevention of thrush is saccharomytes boulardi.

Matching it up

TAKE PROBIOTICS WITH
- Antibiotics

DON'T TAKE PROBIOTICS WITH
- No known interactions

When should I take my supplement?

Probiotics should ideally be taken thirty minutes to one hour before or two hours after a meal to avoid the high acid environment of the stomach at meal times. When using with antibiotics, supplements should be taken during the course of antibiotics one hour away from the antibiotic dose and probiotic supplementation should be continued for at least two weeks after finishing the course of antibiotics.

What happens if I take too much?

No toxicity symptoms have been seen in healthy individuals.

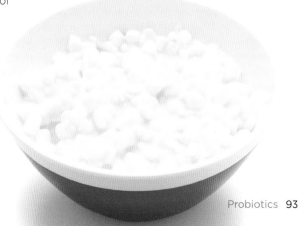

Glucosamine

The Snapshot

Glucosamine is found in all human and animal cartilage as well as the fluid surrounding the joints and helps keep the joint strong and healthy. Supplements are available in the form of glucosamine sulphate and glucosamine hydrochloride, and are recommended for those suffering osteoarthritis or brittle joints. Glucosamine is considered a safe nutrient and no toxicity symptoms have been recognized however those with diabetes should consult their doctor before taking. Glucosamine is also not recommended during pregnancy and breastfeeding, and those with a shellfish allergy should avoid supplements derived from this source.

What does it do?

It plays a role in the formation and repair of cartilage, helping to keep joints healthy.

How do I know if I'm deficient?

As glucosamine is naturally produced by the body, it is not classed as an essential nutrient therefore there are no recognised deficiency signs and symptoms. However, due to its role in cartilage repair, osteoarthritis, sore and brittle joints can result from long-term wear and tear combined with a lack of glucosamine to repair the tissue.

What foods does it come in?

Glucosamine is found in all forms of healthy cartilage such as the outer shell of crustaceans such as lobster and crab as well as animal joints. Most supplements are derived from these sources, direct consumption of these foods is not recommended.

Is a supplement recommended for me?

There have been many studies looking at the effectiveness of glucosamine as a treatment for osteoarthritis and brittle joints. Some studies show pain relief similar to other pharmaceutical anti-inflammatories and others indicate it to be no better than a placebo. However, all studies do indicate that glucosamine is most effective when taken in the initial stages of mild to moderate osteoarthritis or brittle joints. Therefore it is recommended to begin supplementing at the first signs of joint degeneration.

Is a supplement recommended for me?

There are two forms of glucosamine widely available on the market. These are glucosamine sulphate and glucosamine hydrochloride. Glucosamine hydrochloride is the most stable form of the glucosamine, however glucosamine sulphate is the most widely studied. Sulphate also plays a role in joint health so it's believed that this may help contribute to joint repair, however there are no studies to confirm this. Glucosamine sulphate is only stable when combined with potassium or sodium chloride, therefore most supplements using this form will provide glucosamine sulphate potassium chloride complex. Be sure to check the exact amount of glucosamine sulphate the product provides from the potassium chloride complex as sometimes this will not be listed on the packaging and the amount of glucosamine sulphate provided by these complexes can vary. There has been no discernable difference in the effectiveness of either form as long as the therapeutic dose is consumed.

How much should I have?

Glucosamine is not classed as an essential nutrient therefore there is no RDI or AI.

THERAPEUTIC ADULT DOSE

The therapeutic adult dose of glucosamine is **1500mg** per day.

When should I take my supplement?

Glucosamine can be taken with or without food. For those with a sensitive stomach or ulcers, taking glucosamine with food may be beneficial.

Matching it up

TAKE GLUCOSAMINE WITH

- Glucosamine is naturally found with chondroitin, which also supports joint health, so taking these together may provide additional benefit.

DON'T TAKE GLUCOSAMINE WITH

- Although evidence is unclear, caution is advised for diabetics as glucosamine is an amino sugar. Those taking warfarin should also consult with their doctor before commencing glucosamine supplementation. Due to lack of evidence, glucosamine is not recommended during pregnancy or breastfeeding.

What happens if I take too much?

Glucosamine is considered a safe nutrient and symptoms of toxicity have not been established. However taking above the therapeutic dose is not recommended.

What's best for me?

We all have varying nutritional needs at different ages and stages. Make sure you fill your diet with plenty of foods providing the most important nutrients for whatever stage you and your family are at.

Toddlers and Kids (2 + years)

Most important nutrients to include in your diet

- Vitamin A - for cell growth and development
- Calcium - for bone growth and strength
- Vitamin D - for bone growth and strength
- The B group Vitamins - for growth and energy
- Iron - for growth and development
- Omega 3 DHA - for brain health
- Probiotics - for immune system and allergy

DAILY SUPPLEMENT RECOMMENDATIONS
For 'fussy' eaters where dietary intake is lacking

- A good chewable kids multivitamin, as chosen using our guidelines – 1 x per day
- Omega 3 fish oil – containing 100 – 500mg DHA

For those lacking appetite

- A tonic providing iron and B vitamins can be beneficial

For those with eczema/allergy or weakened immune system

- A probiotic powder containing a blend of
- 3 – 6 Billion Lactobacillus acidophilus or Lactobacillus rhamnosus
- 3 – 6 Billion Bifiobacterium

Male – the teenage years

Most important nutrients to include in your diet

- Vitamin A – for cell growth and development
- The B group Vitamins – for growth and energy
- Magnesium – for strong muscle development
- Zinc – for hormonal balance, particularly important if hormonal acne is an issue
- Omega 3 – Fish oil beneficial for those studying, to help support brain health

DAILY SUPPLEMENT RECOMMENDATIONS
For general health where dietary intake is lacking

- A good multivitamin, as chosen using our guidelines – 1 x per day

If experiencing muscle cramps

- 50 – 100mg magnesium – 3 x per day

If experiencing teenage acne

- 12mg zinc – 1 x per day

To help optimize learning and brain health

- 1000mg fish oil – 3 x per day

Female – the teenage years

Most important nutrients to include in your diet

- Vitamin A – for cell growth and development
- The B group vitamins – for growth and energy
- Calcium – for strong bone development
- Iron – for growth and development
- Zinc – for hormonal acne
- Omega 3 – fish oil to help support brain health as well as being an anti inflammatory to assist with period pain.
- Additional vitamin B6 may also be helpful for hormonal support

DAILY SUPPLEMENT RECOMMENDATIONS
For general health where dietary intake may be lacking

- A good multivitamin, as chosen using our guidelines – 1 x per day

If experiencing teenage acne

- 12mg zinc – 1 x per day

To optimize learning and brain health

- 1000mg fish oil – 3 x per day

For mild menstrual symptoms

- 50mg B6 – 1 x per day

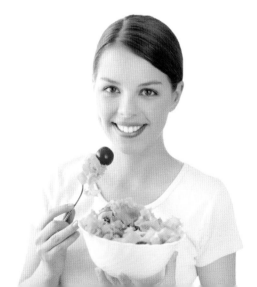

Male in your 20s

Most important nutrients to include in your diet

- The B group vitamins – for stress management and energy
- Magnesium – for muscle and heart health
- Zinc – for hormonal balance
- Coenzyme Q10 – to support energy and heart health
- Omega 3 – to help support brain health, energy and heart health.

DAILY SUPPLEMENT RECOMMENDATIONS

For general health where dietary intake may be lacking
- A good multivitamin, as chosen using our guidelines – 1 x per day

If experiencing muscle cramps
- 50 – 100mg magnesium – 3 x per day

If experiencing hormonal acne
- 12mg zinc – 1 x per day

To optimize learning and brain health
- 1000mg fish oil – 3 x per day

In times of increased stress or fatigue
- B complex – 1 x per day

To support energy production, particularly during sporting activities
- 100mg co enzymeQ10 – 1 x per day

Female in your 20s

Most important nutrients to include in your diet

- The B group vitamins – for stress management and energy
- Calcium – for maintenance of bone health
- Iron – to support healthy blood cells
- Folate – for reproductive health
- Omega 3 – to help support brain health, energy and heart health as well as helping to maintain skin softness and suppleness.

DAILY SUPPLEMENT RECOMMENDATIONS

For general health where dietary intake may be lacking
- A good multivitamin, as chosen using our guidelines – 1 x per day

In times of increased stress or fatigue
- B complex – 1 x per day

For those with heavy menstrual bleeding or low dietary intake of iron
- 5 – 24mg Iron – 1 x per day

For mild menstrual symptoms
- 50mg – 100mg B6 – 1 x per day

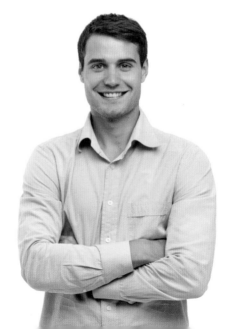

Male in your 30s

Most important nutrients to include in your diet

- The B group vitamins – for stress management and energy
- Magnesium – for muscle and heart health
- Zinc – for reproductive health
- Coenzyme Q10 – to support energy and heart health and impart antioxidant activity to help slow the aging process and support reproductive health
- Omega 3 – to help support brain health, energy and heart health

DAILY SUPPLEMENT RECOMMENDATIONS

For general health where dietary intake may be lacking
- A good multivitamin, as chosen using our guidelines – 1 x per day

If experiencing muscle cramps
- 50 – 100mg magnesium – 3 x per day

If experiencing hormonal acne
- 12mg zinc – 1 x per day

To optimize brain health and for those with family history of heart disease
- 1000 – 2000mg fish oil – 3 x per day

In times of increased stress or fatigue
- B complex – 1 x per day

To support energy production, and for those with family history of heart disease
- 50 – 100mg coenzyme Q10 – 1 x per day

Female in your 30s

Most important nutrients to include in your diet

- The B group vitamins – for stress management and energy
- Calcium – for bone health
- Vitamin D – for bone health
- Iron – to support healthy blood cells
- Folate – for reproductive health
- Coenzyme Q10 – to support energy and heart health, impart antioxidant activity to help slow the aging process and support reproductive health
- Omega 3 – beneficial to help support brain and heart health as well as promoting soft supple skin

DAILY SUPPLEMENT RECOMMENDATIONS

For general health where dietary intake may be lacking
- A good multivitamin, as chosen using our guidelines – 1 x per day

In times of increased stress or fatigue
- B complex – 1 x per day

For those with heavy menstrual bleeding or low dietary intake of iron
- 5 – 24mg iron – 1 x per day

To help support energy and anti-aging
- 50 – 100mg coenzyme Q10 – 1 x per day

To optimize brain and heart health and help keep skin soft and supple
- 1000 – 2000mg fish oil – 3 x per day

Male in your 40s

Most important nutrients to include in your diet

- The B group vitamins – for stress management and energy
- Magnesium – for muscle and heart health
- Zinc – for reproductive and prostate health
- Selenium and vitamin E – to help support prostate health
- Coenzyme Q10 – to support energy, heart health and provide antioxidant activity to help slow the aging process and support reproductive health
- Omega 3 – to help support brain and heart health

DAILY SUPPLEMENT RECOMMENDATIONS

For general health where dietary intake may be lacking

- A good multivitamin, as chosen using our guidelines – 1 x per day

If experiencing muscle cramps

- 50-100mg magnesium – 3 x per day

For prostate and reproductive health

- 12mg zinc – 1 x per day

To optimize brain health and for those with family history of heart disease

- 1000 – 2000mg fish oil – 3 x per day

In times of increased stress or fatigue

- B complex – 1 x per day

To support energy production, and for those with family history of heart disease

- 100mg coenzyme Q10 – 1 x per day

To support healthy joints

- 1500mg glucosamine – 1 x per day

To boost antioxidant activity, cancer prevention and prostate health

- Therapeutic doses of selenium, vitamin A, C & E

Female in your 40s

Most important nutrients to include in your diet

- The B group vitamins – to support stress management and energy
- Calcium – for bone health
- Vitamin D – for bone and general health
- Iron – to support healthy blood cells
- Coenzyme Q10 – to boost antioxidant activity, helping to slow the signs of aging and support energy and heart health
- Omega 3 – to help support brain and heart health
- Antioxidant nutrients for anti-aging activity

DAILY SUPPLEMENT RECOMMENDATIONS

For general health where dietary intake may be lacking

- A good multivitamin, as chosen using our guidelines – 1 x per day

In times of increased stress or fatigue

- B Complex – 1 x per day

For those with heavy menstrual bleeding or low dietary intake of iron

- 5 – 24mg iron – 1 x per day

For those with low dietary calcium intake

- 400 – 600mg calcium – 1-2 x per day

To help support energy and anti-aging

- 100mg coenzyme Q10 – 1 x per day

To optimize brain and heart health and help keep skin soft and supple

- 1000 – 2000mg fish oil – 3 x per day

To boost antioxidant/anti-aging activity and cancer prevention

- Therapeutic doses of selenium, vitamin A, C & E

Male in your 50s

Most important nutrients to include in your diet

- The B group vitamins – for stress management and energy
- Magnesium – for muscle and heart health
- Vitamin A, C, E and zinc – for reproductive and prostate health, prevention of Macular degeneration and antioxidant/anti-aging support
- Glucosamine – to support healthy joints
- Antioxidant nutrients – additional support for prostate health and anti-aging benefits
- Coenzyme Q10 – to support energy and heart health and provide antioxidant activity
- Omega 3 - to help support brain and heart health and can act as an anti inflammatory to help reduce possible joint pain

DAILY SUPPLEMENT RECOMMENDATIONS

For general health where dietary intake may be lacking
- A good multivitamin, as chosen using our guidelines – 1 x per day

If experiencing muscle cramps
- 50-100mg magnesium – 3 x per day

For prostate and reproductive health
- 12mg zinc – 1 x per day

To optimize brain and heart health and provide arthritic pain relief
- 1000 – 2000mg fish oil – 3 x per day

In times of increased stress or fatigue
- B complex – 1 x per day

To support energy production, and for those with family history of heart disease
- 100mg coenzyme Q10 – 1 x per day

To support healthy joints
- 1500mg glucosamine – 1 x per day

To boost antioxidant activity, cancer prevention and prostate health
- Therapeutic doses of selenium, vitamin A, C & E

Female in your 50s

Most important nutrients to include in your diet

- Calcium – for bone health
- Vitamin D – for bone health
- The B group Vitamins – for stress management and energy
- Vitamin A, C, E and zinc – for prevention of Macular degeneration and antioxidant/anti-aging support
- Glucosamine – to support healthy joints
- Coenzyme Q10 – to boost antioxidant activity, helping to slow the signs of aging and support energy and heart health
- Omega 3 – to help support brain and heart health
- The antioxidant nutrients – for added antioxidant/anti-aging activity

DAILY SUPPLEMENT RECOMMENDATIONS

For general health where dietary intake may be lacking
- A good multivitamin, as chosen using our guidelines – 1 x per day
- 400-600mg calcium – 1–2 x per day
- Vitamin D3 1000IU

In times of increased stress or fatigue
- B complex – 1 x per day

To help support energy and anti-aging
- 100mg coenzyme Q10 – 1 x per day

To optimize brain and heart health and help keep skin soft and supple
- 1000-2000mg fish oil – 3 x per day

To boost antioxidant/anti-aging activity and cancer prevention
- Therapeutic doses of selenium, vitamin A, C & E

Male 60 +

Most important nutrients to include in your diet

- The B group Vitamins – for stress management and energy
- Folate – to support cardiovascular health
- Vitamin A, C, E and zinc – for reproductive and prostate health, prevention of Macular degeneration and antioxidant/anti-aging support
- Glucosamine – to support healthy joints
- Calcium – for bone health
- Vitamin D3 – for bone health
- Coenzyme Q10 – to support energy and heart health and provide antioxidant activity
- Magnesium – for muscle and heart health
- Omega 3 – to help support brain and heart health and can act as an anti inflammatory to help reduce possible joint pain
- Antioxidant nutrients – for added antioxidant/anti-aging activity

DAILY SUPPLEMENT RECOMMENDATIONS

For general health where dietary intake may be lacking

- A good multivitamin, as chosen using our guidelines – 1 x per day
- 1500mg glucosamine – 1 x per day

For heart healthy and if experiencing muscle cramps

- 50–100mg magnesium – 3 x per day

For prostate and reproductive health

- 12mg zinc – 1 x per day

To optimize brain and heart health and provide arthritic pain relief

- 1000 – 2000mg fish oil – 3 x per day

To support energy production, and for those with family history of heart disease

- 100mg coenzyme Q10 – 1 x per day

To boost antioxidant activity for cancer prevention, prostate health and prevention of Macular degeneration

- Therapeutic doses of selenium, vitamin A, C & E

For bone health if dietary intake is lacking

- 600mg calcium – 1 x per day
- 1000IU vitamin D – 1 x per day

Female 60 +

Most important nutrients to include in your diet

- Calcium – for bone health
- Vitamin D – for bone health
- Glucosamine – to support healthy joints
- The B group Vitamins – for stress management and energy
- Vitamin A, C, E and Zinc – for prevention of Macular degeneration and antioxidant/anti-aging support
- Coenzyme Q10 – to boost antioxidant activity, helping to slow the signs of aging and support energy and heart health
- Omega 3 – to help support brain and heart health
- Added antioxidant nutrients such as selenium can also be useful for further antioxidant/anti-aging activity

DAILY SUPPLEMENT RECOMMENDATIONS

For general health where dietary intake may be lacking

- A good multivitamin, as chosen using our guidelines – 1 x per day
- 1500mg glucosamine – 1 x per day

To support bone health where dietary intake may be lacking

- 400 – 600mg calcium – 1–2 x per day
- Vitamin D3 1000IU

To help support heart health, energy and anti-aging

- 100mg coenzyme Q10 – 1 x per day

To optimize brain and heart health, help relieve arthritis and help keep skin soft and supple

- 1000 – 2000mg fish oil – 3 x per day

To boost antioxidant activity for anti-aging benefits, cancer prevention and prevention of Macular Degeneration

- Therapeutic doses of selenium, vitamin A, C & E

Male wishing to conceive

Most important nutrients to include in your diet

- Zinc – for testosterone metabolism, sperm production, sperm motility and sperm count
- B6 – works together with zinc for sperm production
- Folate and vitamin B12 – work together for sperm production, sperm motility and sperm count and required for the synthesis of the genetic code (DNA and RNA)
- Vitamin A, C and E – provides antioxidant activity to help improve sperm quality
- Manganese – involved in testosterone production. Deficiency is linked to infertility, low sex drive and low sperm count
- Co Q10 – large amounts can be found in seminal fluid. Supports energy production and provides antioxidant activity
- Omega 3 DHA – improves sperm quality and motility
- Carnitine – helps improve sperm maturation and motility as well as providing antioxidant activity
- L-arginine – helps stimulate sperm motility

DAILY SUPPLEMENT RECOMMENDATIONS
Look for a multivitamin which provides

- Zinc – 10 – 30mg per day
- Vitamin B6 – 2 – 20mg per day
- Folate (ideally as calcium folinate) - 400mcg per day
- Vitamin B12 – 10 – 50mcg per day
- Vitamin A – 1000 – 1500mcg per day
- Vitamin C – 100 – 500mg per day
- Vitamin E – 10 – 50mg per day
- Manganese – 1 – 5mcg per day

For additional support

- Co Q10 – 30 – 100mg per day
- DHA – 200 – 2000mg/day
- Carnitine – 1000 – 3000mg/day
- L-Arginine – 1000 – 3000mg/day

Female wishing to conceive

Most important nutrients to include in your diet

- Folate – for healthy development of the neural tube
- Choline – for healthy development of the neural tube and brain development
- Iodine – for brain development and prevention of intellectual impairment
- Iron – For fetal growth and development
- Biotin – for brain and tissue development
- Vitamin B12 – for production of DNA and RNA for cell division and growth
- Vitamin D – for growth and bone development
- Calcium – for growth and bone development
- Coenzyme Q10 – for antioxidant activity to support egg health
- Vitamin B6 – to support hormone balance
- Zinc – to support ovulation

DAILY SUPPLEMENT RECOMMENDATIONS
Look for a preconception/pregnancy multivitamin that provides

- Folate (ideally as calcium follinate) – 500mcg per day
- Choline – 500mg per day
- Iodine – 250mcg per day
- Iron – 5 – 24mg per day (iron levels should be monitored for individual requirements)
- Biotin – 300mcg per day
- Vitamin B12 – 500mcg per day
- Vitamin D – 1000IU per day
- Calcium – 100-120mg per day (ideally balanced with magnesium in a 2:1 ratio)

Additional support for healthy eggs

- Co enzyme Q10 – 30 – 100mg
- DHA – 200 – 2000mg

Pregnant female

Most important nutrients to include in your diet

- Folate – for healthy development of the neural tube
- Choline – for healthy development of the neural tube and brain development
- Iodine – for brain development and prevention of intellectual impairment
- Iron – For fetal growth and development
- Biotin – for brain and tissue development
- Vitamin B12 – for production of DNA and RNA to support cell division and growth
- Vitamin D – for growth and bone development
- Calcium – for growth and bone development
- Omega 3 DHA – is an important component of all cell membranes and can assist in the prevention of postpartum depression

DAILY SUPPLEMENT RECOMMENDATIONS

A good broad spectrum pregnancy/ preconception multivitamin should provide good nutritional support during this time. Look for one that includes

- Folate (ideally as calcium folinate) – 500mcg per day
- Choline – 450 – 500mg per day
- Iodine – 250mcg per day
- Iron – 12 – 24mg per day
- Biotin – 300mcg
- Vitamin B12 – 500mcg per day
- Vitamin D – 1000IU
- Calcium – 100 – 120mg (ideally balanced with Magnesium in a 2:1 ratio)

An additional supplement of DHA for brain development and prevention of postpartum depression is also a beneficial addition. This should ideally be taken as a separate supplement to your multivitamin

- DHA – 200 – 2000mg per day

Breastfeeding female

Most important nutrients to include in your diet

- Choline – for healthy brain development and support of long term learning and memory
- Omega 3 DHA – is an important component of all cell membranes and can assist in the prevention of postpartum depression
- Iodine – for brain development and prevention of intellectual impairment
- Folate – to support healthy brain development
- Iron – to support infant growth and development
- Biotin – for brain and tissue development
- Vitamin B12 – for production of DNA and RNA to support growth and development
- Vitamin D – for growth and bone development
- Calcium – for growth and bone development

DAILY SUPPLEMENT RECOMMENDATIONS

Look for a pregnancy/breastfeeding multivitamin providing

- Choline – 450 – 500mg per day
- Calcium folinate – 400 – 500mcg per day
- Iodine – 250mcg per day
- Iron – 5 – 12mg per day (depending on individual requirements)
- Biotin – 300mcg per day
- Vitamin D – 500IU – 1000IU per day
- Calcium – 100–120mg per day (ideally balanced with Magnesium in a 2:1 ratio)

An additional supplement for DHA brain development and prevention of postpartum depression is also recommended. This should ideally be taken as a separate supplement to your multivitamin

- DHA – 200 – 2000mg per day

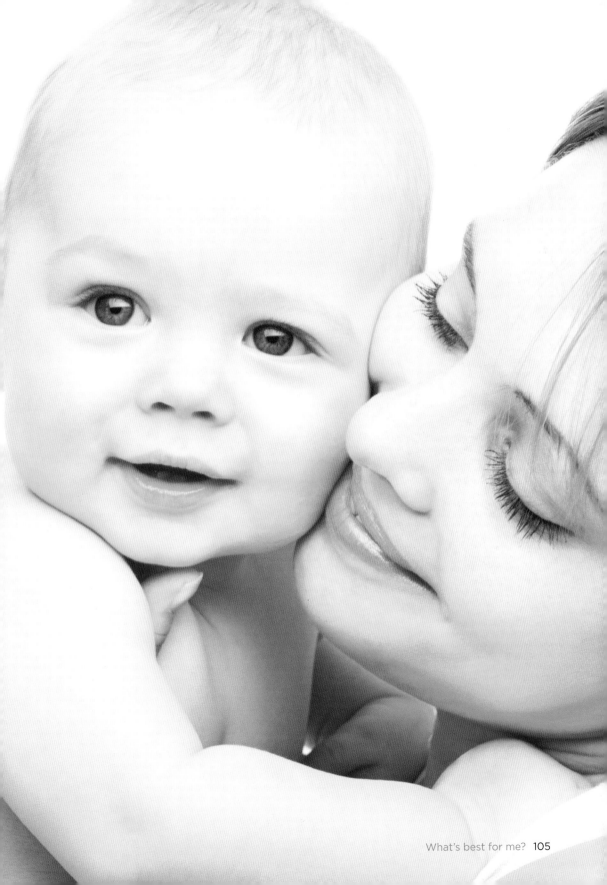

Recipes

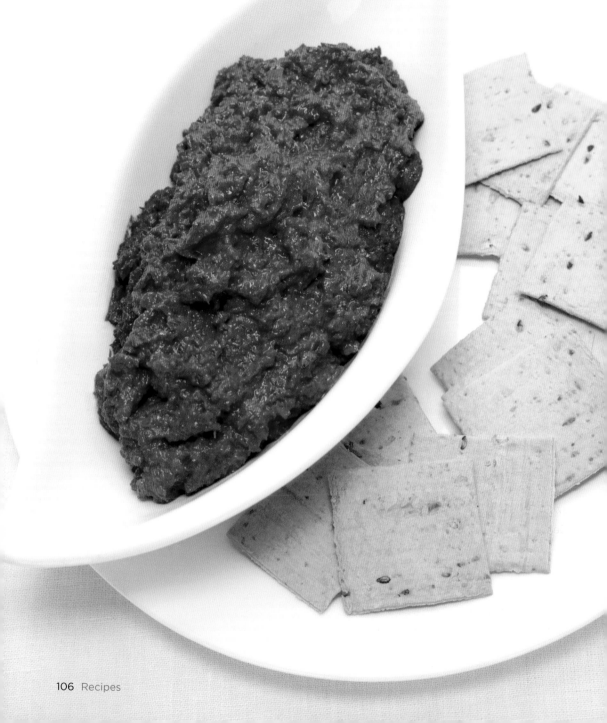

Mains

Beetroot Dip

Packed with antioxidants this simple dish is a great, easy way to boost your nutrient intake. Enjoy with sliced carrot and celery, crackers or spread on a sandwich.

Ingredients

500g tin of baby beetroot (or cook your own!)
3/4 cup greek style natural yoghurt
1 tablespoon lemon juice

Method

Put all ingredients into a blender or food processor, whizz and you're done!

Cheesy baked Eggplant with Tofu

Ingredients

1 large eggplant, thinly sliced
1/4 cup extra virgin olive oil
200g firm tofu, thinly sliced
1/4 cup chopped fresh oregano, basil and parsley
500mg tomato sugo
2 cloves garlic, crushed
1/3 cup grated tasty or cheddar cheese
1/4 cup finely grated parmesan
Sea salt and fresh ground black pepper

Method

Preheat oven to 180° C

Spread eggplant slices onto a large tray and sprinkle with salt on both sides. Leave for about 30 minutes or until moisture beads appear. Rinse thoroughly under cold water and pat dry.

Brush a large baking tray with olive oil and spread the eggplant slices over the tray. Drizzle with extra olive oil and bake in the oven for 15-20 minutes or until golden brown.

Combine tomato sugo, garlic and remaining oregano, basil and parsley mix into a bowl and season with salt and pepper, set aside.

Place 1/2 the eggplant slices, into the base of a large baking dish, overlapping slightly to fully cover the base. Top with slices of the tofu and half of the oregano, basil and parsley mix.

Layer the remaining eggplant over the tofu layer. Poor the tomato sugo mix over the final eggplant layer and sprinkle with the cheeses. Bake for 35 minutes or until cheese is melted and golden.

Slice into 4 large slices and serve with spinach salad (optional)

Serves 4

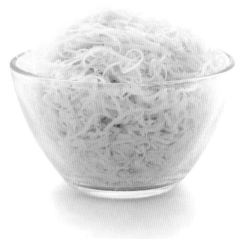

Chicken and Roasted Almond Stir-fry

Stir fry's make a lovely, simple, nutrient packed mid week meal. Enjoy!

Ingredients
1/4 cup almonds
2 tbsp peanut or olive oil
750g free range chicken breast, cut into strips
2 red onions, thinly sliced
1 red capsicum
200g broccoli, cut into bite size pieces
2 tbsp salt reduced soy sauce
2 tbsp rice wine vinegar (or another 2 tbsp soy sauce)
1 tbsp oyster sauce
5 spring onions, sliced diagonally
Cracked black pepper

Method
Heat 1 tbsp oil in the wok or large fry pan, when hot, roast the almonds for 2 – 3 minutes or until golden then set aside. Add additional tbsp oil if required. Add chicken to the pan and cook for 3 – 5 minutes until lightly browned all over, set aside. Add the onion, capsicum and broccoli to the pan and cook over medium heat for 4 – 5 minutes or until vegetables have softened slightly. Increase the heat and add the soy sauce, rice wine vinegar and oyster sauce. Toss the vegetables well through the sauce and bring to the boil. Return the chicken to the pan and cook over high heat for 1 – 2 minutes to make sure chicken is entirely cooked through. Season with cracked black pepper to taste. Stir through the almonds and spring onion and serve piping hot!

Chicken on a bed of spicy lentils

Ingredients
Extra virgin olive oil
1 onion, diced
1 clove garlic, grated
2 tsp harissa paste
1 tsp ground coriander
1 tsp ground cumin
125g (2/3 cup) green lentils
500ml (2 cups) chicken or vegetable stock
125ml (1/2 cup) tomato sugo
sea salt and fresh ground pepper
4 Chicken breasts
1/4 cup chopped coriander

Method
Heat a medium-sized saucepan over a medium-high heat. Add a splash of oil and cook the onion for 3 – 4 minutes. Add the garlic, harissa, coriander and cumin. Cook for a further 1 – 2 minutes, stirring often. Add lentils, stock and tomato sugo, and bring to the boil. Reduce the heat and cook for 45 minutes, stirring occasionally, until the lentils are cooked and the sauce is reduced. Season to taste.

Heat a heavy-based frypan over a medium-high heat. Add a splash of oil and cook the chicken on each side until golden brown cooked through. Check seasoning on the lentils and stir through coriander leaves.

Spoon the lentils into serving bowls, or one large platter. Slice the chicken diagonally and layer across lentils. Serve immediately.

Serves 4 - 6

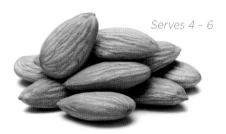

Chicken fajitas

Ingredients

500g skinless chicken breast fillets
2 red onions, sliced
1 tbsp oil
1 tsp paprika
1/2 tsp ground cumin
1/2 tsp ground coriander
Juice of 3 large limes or lemons
1/4 tsp chilli powder
1/2 red capsicum, diced
2 tomatoes diced
400g can cannellini beans, drained and rinsed
2 tbsp chopped parsley
1 small red chilli, deseeded and diced
2 cups lettuce, shredded
150mg natural yoghurt
150g grated cheddar cheese
Sea salt and fresh ground pepper
8 warm tortillas or pitas

Method

Preheat oven to 180º C.

Slice the chicken fillets into 1cm wide strips and place in a bowl. Combine the oil, paprika, cumin, coriander, chilli powder and 1/2 the lemon or lime juice and pour over chicken. Stir through and allow to marinate for 5 – 30 minutes.

Place the diced capsicum, tomatoes, chilli and cannellini beans in a bowl. Add the rest of the lemon or lime juice and parsley and season with salt and pepper to taste. Set aside until ready to serve.

Heat a heavy based fry pan over medium to high heat. Add the chicken and any surplus marinade to the pan and cook until golden brown.

Warm the tortillas or pitas in the preheated oven for a few minutes then place on a plate and serve with the lettuce, chicken, bean mix, cheese and yoghurt, allowing everyone to make up their own.

Serves 4

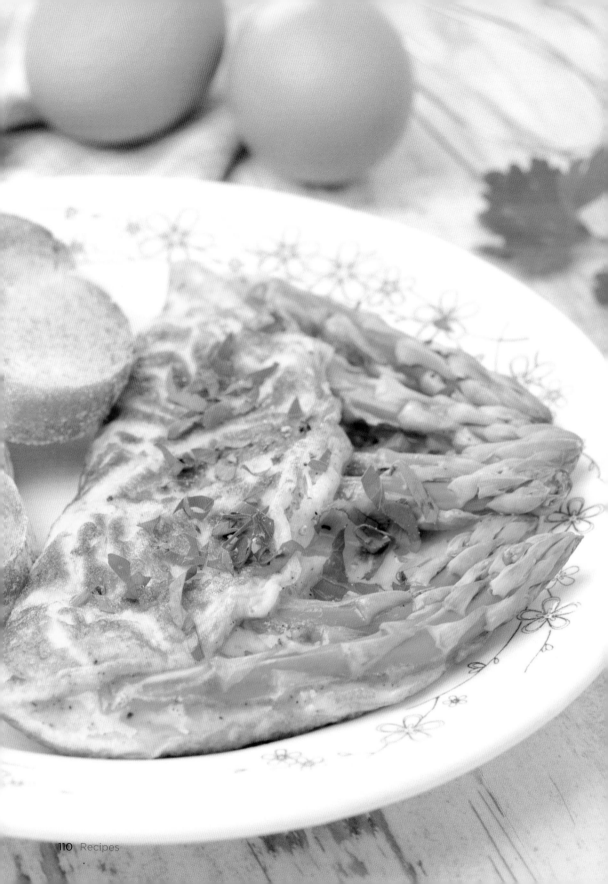

Easy Asparagus Omelette

Ingredients

15 asparagus spears, ends trimmed
12 free range eggs
Freshly ground black pepper
1 tbsp unsalted butter
500g parmasen cheese, shaved into thin slices

Method

Cut the asparagus spears into 5cm lengths and slice in half any thicker stems. Cook the asparagus in the boiling water for 30 seconds to 1 minute or until it turns bright green. Drain and transfer to a large bowl of iced water until cool. Drain.

Preheat grill to 220 degrees Celcius. Whisk eggs and pepper in a large bowl to blend well. Melt butter in a large non-stick ovenproof sauté pan over medium heat, swirling the pan to coat all sides with butter.

Add eggs and then asparagus to the pan. Gently stir to lift the cooked egg from the bottom of the pan and stir it into the uncooked portion, be cautious not to over-stir. As the omelette begins to set give it a final gentle stir. Scatter cheese over the top.

Put the pan under the pre heated grill and cook for 1 minute or until the omelette has set and the cheese has melted. Serve on wholemeal toast and fresh baby spinach.

Easy Lamb Stew

A hearty, nourishing dish for Mum, bub and the whole family. This easy meal can even be blended up and enjoyed by your little one, 6 months plus!

Ingredients

1 tablespoon olive oil
2 cloves garlic, crushed or finely grated
1 large brown onion, chopped
2 carrots, sliced
2 sticks celery, sliced
500g lamb shoulder, diced
1 litre, low salt chicken or vegetable stock
2 x 400g can diced tomatoes
2 x 400g can chickpeas (or mixed beans if preferred)
1/2 cup flat leaf parsley, chopped

Method

Heat oil in a deep saucepan over medium heat. Add garlic and onion, cook for 2 – 3 minutes. Add carrot and celery and stir well for 3 – 4 minutes until onion has softened. Add the lamb, stock and tomatoes and bring to the boil. Reduce the heat and simmer covered for 1 hour or until lamb is tender. Or transfer to a slow cooker and allow to cook on low. Stir in parsley before serving.

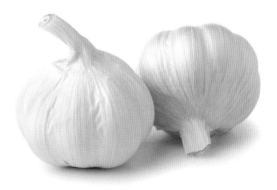

Fish with Ginger and Coriander

This is a super tasty, easy dish and the ginger is great for a queasy pregnant stomach!

Ingredients

1 tbsp peanut oil
1 red onion, finely sliced
3 tsps ground coriander
500g firm white fish (such as rockling), diced into 2cm cubes
1 tbsp fresh ginger, finely sliced
1 green chilli, deseeded and finely sliced
2 tbsp lime juice
1/4 coriander leaves, roughly chopped

Method

Heat the oil in a wok over high heat, add the onion and stir fry for 3 – 4 minutes until soft and lightly golden. Add the ground coriander, stirring frequently. Cook for 1 – 2 minutes until fragrant. Add the fish, ginger and chilli and stir fry for around 5 minutes or until fish is completely cooked through. Stir through the lime juice and coridander and serve with some steaming jasmine rice.

Indian Chicken Quinoa

Quinoa is a nutrient packed 'supergrain' and makes a great addition to any diet, especially during pregnancy and breastfeeding. But what do you do with it? Here's a tasty, easy recipe for all to enjoy!

Ingredients

2 tbsp sesame or olive oil
1 tbs black mustard seeds
6 - 8 dried curry leaves
2 tsp garam masala
3 green chillies, deseeded and finely sliced
1 onion, finely chopped
1 1/2 cups quinoa
1/2 cup yellow split peas
3 cups chicken stock (salt reduced)
1 1/2 cups shredded cooked chicken
80g baby spinach leaves

Method

Heat oil in a large pan over medium heat. Add the mustard seeds and cook until they start to pop. Add the curry leaves, garam marsala, chilli, onion and cook for 4 – 5 minutes or until golden and fragrant. Add quinoa and split peas and stir well to coat. Add stock, bring to the boil and simmer over low heat for 25 minutes, add chicken and spinach and stir until wilted and heated through. Season to taste and enjoy!

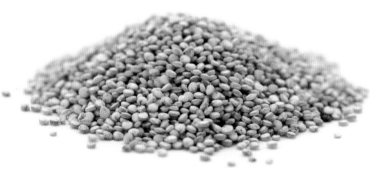

Lamburgers!

Although you can use beef in these tasty burgers, lamb adds a tasty twist on the Aussie hamburger.

Ingredients

500g lean lamb mince
1 onion, finely chopped
1 clove garlic, crushed
2 tbsp fresh mint, chopped (or 2 tsp dried)
2 tbsp fresh oregano, chopped (or 2 tsp dried)
1 tbsp lemon juice
Sea salt and craked pepper
1/4 cup fetta cheese, crumbled
Plain flour
Olive oil for the grill

Method

In a large bowl, mix the lamb, onion, mint, oregano, lemon juice and season with salt and pepper. Mix with your hands until well combined. Separate into balls, coat your hands with plain flour and press flat with your hands to form patties. Drizzle some olive oil in a pre-heated grill or BBQ plate. Cook for 5 minutes or until nicely golden brown on the bottom, flip and place a portion of feta on the cooked side. Cook for another 5 – 10 minutes or until well done. Serve on fresh buns with tomatoes, spinach and cheese. Enjoy!

Moroccan Spiced Fish Stew

This delicious winter warming dish is one of my favourites! A dinner staple in our house. Packs a flavour punch, full of nutrients and nice and easy too!

Ingredients

1 tbsp olive oil
1 onion, finely diced
1 fennel bulb, finely sliced
1 red chilli, deseeded and diced (leave out if you prefer a milder dish)
1 cloves garlic, grated or crushed
1/2 tsp sweet paprika
1/2 tsp ground coriander
Pinch saffron threads
1 x 400g tin chopped tomatoes
2 bay leaves
1 cup (250ml) fish stock or seasoned water
300g small new potatoes, quartered
500g rockling (or other firm white fish), cubed in 2cm pieces
50g baby spinach leaves
1/4 cup fresh coriander leaves, roughly chopped

Method

Heat oil in a large saucepan over medium heat. Add the onion and fennel and stir for 3 – 4 minutes until softened. Add the chilli, garlic and spices, stirring well for another 1 – 2 minutes until fragrant. Add the tomatoes, bay leaves and stock. Bring to the boil, then add the potatoes and cook for 10 – 15 minutes until potatoes are tender. Add the fish and allow to cook for 5 – 10 minutes until fish is cooked through. Stir through the spinach and coriander until wilted, then serve over steaming rice or cous cous or serve with crusty bread.

Moroccan Spiced Fish Stew

This delicious winter warming dish is one of my favourites! A dinner staple in our house. Packs a flavour punch, full of nutrients and nice and easy too!

Ingredients

1 tbsp olive oil
1 onion, finely diced
1 fennel bulb, finely sliced
1 red chilli, deseeded and diced (leave out if you prefer a milder dish)
1 cloves garlic, grated or crushed
1/2 tsp sweet paprika
1/2 tsp ground coriander
Pinch saffron threads
1 x 400g tin chopped tomatoes
2 bay leaves
1 cup (250ml) fish stock or seasoned water
300g small new potatoes, quartered
500g rockling (or other firm white fish), cubed in 2cm pieces
50g baby spinach leaves
1/4 cup fresh coriander leaves, roughly chopped

Method

Heat oil in a large saucepan over medium heat. Add the onion and fennel and stir for 3 – 4 minutes until softened. Add the chilli, garlic and spices, stirring well for another 1 – 2 minutes until fragrant. Add the tomatoes, bay leaves and stock. Bring to the boil, then add the potatoes and cook for 10 – 15 minutes until potatoes are tender. Add the fish and allow to cook for 5 – 10 minutes until fish is cooked through. Stir through the spinach and coriander until wilted, then serve over steaming rice or cous cous or serve with crusty bread.

Spicy Ratatouille

This dish is surprisingly easy and versatile. Can be served as a main with some crusty bread or alongside some roast meat.

Ingredients

3 tbsp olive oil
2 brown onions, diced
1 medium sweet potato, peeled and diced
1 eggplant, diced
2 red capsicums, seeded and diced
2 large zucchinis, thickly sliced
2 green chillies, sliced (optional)
2 garlic cloves, crushed or grated
2 cans chopped tomatoes
1/3 cup pitted black olives
1 tbsp fresh basil, chopped
1 tbsp fresh parsley, chopped
Freshly cracked pepper
Shaved parmesan to serve

Method

Heat the olive oil in a saucepan over medium heat. Add the onion, sweet potato and cook for 5 minutes or until the onion is soft and golden. Add the garlic and cook for a further 3 minutes. Add the eggplant, red capsicum, green chillis and zucchini and cook for 5 minutes. Add the tomatoes, bring to the boil then cover and simmer for 15 minutes or until the vegetables are almost tender. Season with freshly cracked black pepper to taste. Lift the lid and simmer uncovered for 10 minutes or until vegetables are tender and sauce has reduced. Serve topped with shaved parmesan.

Parsley Pesto

Packed with iron, B12 and antioxidants this versatile dish can be added to soups or salads, spread under bruschetta as a sandwich base.

Ingredients

1 bunch Italian flat leaf parsley
1 clove garlic, peeled and chopped
50g pine nuts
50g parmesan, finely grated
1 lemon rind and juice
150 – 200ml olive oil
Fresh ground black pepper to taste

Method

Place the parsley, garlic, pine nuts, parmesan, lemon rind and juice into a food processor and process until combined. Slowly drizzle in the olive oil until you reach your desired consistency.

Spiced Beef and Lentil Burgers

An excellent source of vitamin B12, iron, choline and protein these tasty burgers make the perfect winter meal. Even if you've never tried lentils, give these a go. You won't even know they're healthy!

Ingredients

500g lean minced beef
400g can lentils, drained and rinsed
1 onion, finely diced
3 sliced of wholegrain bread, crusts removed and torn into small pieces
1 egg
1 tsp ground cumin
1 tsp sweet paprika

Method

Line a baking tray with baking paper. Place the beef, lentils, onion, bread, egg and spices into a bowl. Mix thoroughly until well combined. Shape the mixture into 8 – 10 patties and place on the pre-lined baking tray. Cover with cling wrap and refrigerate for around 30 minutes. Cook on an oiled barbeque grill until cooked through and golden brown.

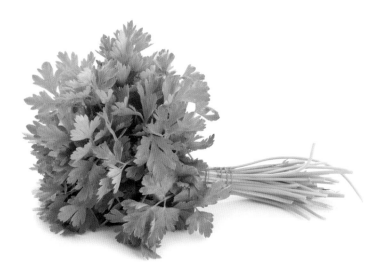

Spinach and Beetroot Salad

Ingredients

3 cups baby spinach leaves
2 whole cooked beetroots, chopped into 2cm chunks
1 baby fennel, thinly sliced
1 stalk celery thinly sliced

Dressing

2 tbsp extra virgin olive oil
1 tbsp lime juice
Sea salt and cracked black pepper
1/2 clove crushed garlic

Method

Wash baby spinach, drain excess moisture and place in large serving bown. Add the beetroot, baby fennel and celery.

To make the dressing mix the olive oil with the lime juice and crushed garlic, season to taste with sea salt and cracked black pepper.

Pour dressing over salad, mixing to combine

Serves 4

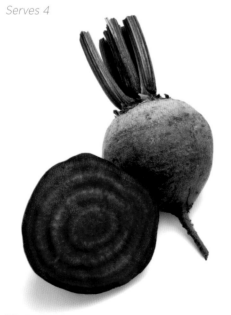

Super Tasty Meatballs in Tomato Sauce

This dish is a crowd pleaser. Perfect for a cosy winter meal. Super tasty, super nutritious and great for the whole family.

Ingredients

500g lean minced beef
70g (1 cup) fresh breadcrumbs
80mls (1/3 cup) skim milk
2 green chillies, deseeded, finely chopped
1 tsp ground cumin
Salt and freshly ground black pepper, to taste
2 x 400g tins chopped tomatoes
2 cloves garlic, crushed
2 tbsp olive oil
3 tbsp parsley, chopped

Method

Place the beef, breadcrumbs, milk, green chillies and cumin in a bowl and mix until thoroughly combined. Season with salt and pepper and roll into small balls (about 1.5cm). Set aside.

For the sauce, place the oil in a wide saucepan over low to medium heat, add the chopped garlic and cook gently for 5 minutes until lightly golden but not brown. Add the chopped tomatoes and simmer gently for 5 minutes. Add the meatballs and continue to simmer for another 10 minutes, turning occasionally, or until cooked through. Stir through the chopped parsley and serve over pasta, cous cous or fresh crusty bread.

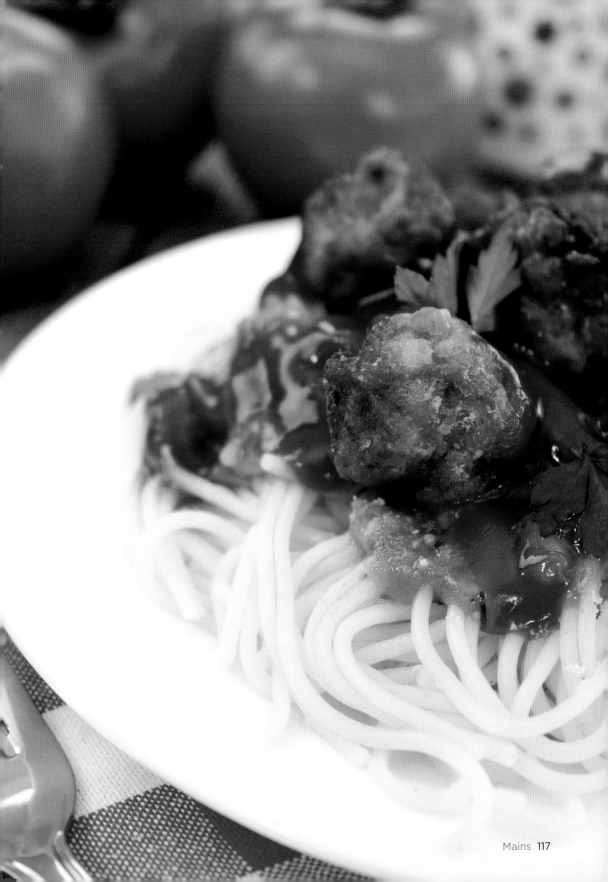

Tasty Pork Stew

Ingredients

1 tbsp olive oil
2 brown onions, chopped
500g lean pork, diced
2 teaspoons sweet paprika
1 tsp hot paprika
1/2 tsp dried thyme
2 tbsp tomato paste
1/4 cup red lentils
1 12 cups beef or vegetable stock
Greek yoghurt and 2 tablespoons of chopped
parsley to serve
Fresh ground black pepper

Method

Heat olive oil in a casserole pot over high heat.
Add the onion, pork sweet and hot paprika
and cook, stirring for 3 - 4 minutes or until
browned. Add the thyme, tomato paste, lentils,
stock and black pepper to taste. Bring to the
boil, then reduce heat to very low and cook,
covered for 20 minutes, stirring occasionally.
Uncover and cook for another 15 – 20 minutes
or until thickened. Serve with a generous dolop
of greek yoghurt and a sprinkle of parsley.

Veggie Croquettes

This fabulous family dish is a great way to
disguise boring veggies!

Ingredients

1 tbsp olive oil plus extra for cooking
300g sweet potato, diced
150g broccoli florets
1 medium onion, diced
1 clove garlic, crushed
75g grated carrot
100g cheddar cheese
Freshly cracked black pepper

Method

Boil or steam potatoes for 15 minutes or until
tender. Boil or steam broccoli for 5 minutes
or until tender. Once cooked, chop broccoli
florets into small pieces.

Sauté the onion and garlic in the olive oil for
2 – 3 minutes or until softened, add the grated
carrot and sauté for a further minute. Mash the
sweet potato with the cheese then mix in the
broccoli, onion, garlic and carrot. Season to
taste with black pepper.

Hand form into small burgers. Add enough oil
to lightly coat a fry pan and cook until golden
brown.

Tuna Casserolet

Ingredients
2 tbsp extra virgin olive oil
1 leek (white part only) thinly sliced
1 carrot, finely chopped
1 celery stalk, finely chopped
400g can chopped tomatoes
2 x 400g can cannellini beans, rinsed
200ml chicken or vegetable stock
1 tbsp Dijon mustard
2 x 200g yellowfin tuna fillets
1 cup (50g) panko breadcrumbs (or
wholmeal dry breadcrumbs)
1 clove garlic, crushed
1 tbsp flat leaf parsley, finely chopped

Method
Heat 1 tbsp of the olive oil in a pan over
medium-low heat. Cook leek, carrot and celery
for 10 minutes, stirring until softened. Add
tomato, beans and stock and simmer over
medium heat for 20 minutes until slightly
reduced, then stir in mustard.

Preheat oven to 200°C. Lightly oil 4 individual
baking dishes or ramekins.
Heat a lightly oiled pan over high heat. Sear
tuna for 1 minute on each side. Cut into bite
sized pieces. Layer beans, then tuna, then
more beans in the dishes.

Lightly mix panko (or wholemeal
breadcrumbs), garlic, parsley and 1 tbsp oil,
then top each dish with the mixture. Place
in the oven a and bake for 20 minutes until
golden brown and bubbling.

Serve immediately with salad

Serves 4

Zucchini and Humus Frittata

Ingredients
1 large zucchini, grated
500g baby spinach leaves
2 tbsp extra virgin olive oil
1 red onion, thinly sliced
1 tbsp chopped basil
1 tbsp chopped parsley
8 organic free range eggs, whisked
1 tsp grated lemon zest
3 tbsp humus
2 tbsp natural low fat yoghurt

Method
Wash zucchini and grate, set aside. Wash
spinach and blanch until wilted. Drain excess
moisture and set aside. Heat oil in a non-
stick 24cm fry pan. Add onion and cook over
medium heat until soft. Add herbs and cook
until wilted. Add zucchini and spinach and
arrange evenly in pan.

Pre heat grill. Whisk together eggs, lemon
zest, hummus and yoghurt and pour over
vegetables. Season with salt and pepper in
desired.

Cook over a medium heat until the base is just
set. Cover frypan handle in foil and transfer
pan to the preheated frill and cook until set
and golden brown.

Cut 4 large slices and serve immediately with
salad.

Serves 4

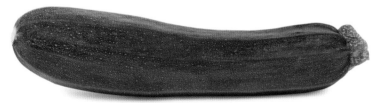

Soups

Cauliflower and Walnut Soup

Cauliflower is a good source of choline, which is essential for healthy brain development. Combined with walnuts, this makes a delicious winter warming soup.

Ingredients

1 cauliflower, cut into florets
1 onion, chopped
500ml vegetable stock
2 cups skim mik
3 tbsp walnuts, lightly broken
River or sea salt and freshly ground black pepper
Sweet paprika for garnish

Method

Place the cauliflower florets, onion and stock in a large saucepan over high heat. Bring to the boil, cover and simmer for about 15 minutes or until cauliflower is tender. Add the skim milk and walnuts then blend with a hand held blender or food processor until smooth. Season to taste and garnish with a sprinkling of sweet paprika.

Creamy Mushroom Soup

This easy dish is a family favourite and always pleases at dinner parties! It's also packed with nutrients including all important vitamin B12 and vitamin D.

Ingredients

15g butter
1 red onion, finely chopped
450g button mushrooms, finely chopped
300ml vegetable stock
300ml low fat milk
1 - 2 tbsp fresh tarragon, chopped
Freshly ground black pepper

Method

Melt the butter in a large pan, add the red onion and cook over a low heat for 5 minutes. Add the mushrooms and cook for a further 3 minutes, stirring gently. Add the stock and the milk and bring to the boil. Cover and simmer gently for about 20 minutes until the mushrooms are tender. Add the tarragon and stir through, season to taste with black pepper. Blend the soup with a hand blender or food processor. Serve topped with some fresh tarragon leaves.

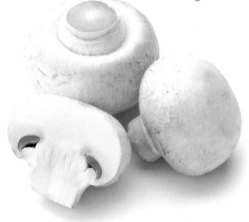

Broccoli and Almond Soup

Super easy, super tasty and super healthy!
I always have some of this delicious soup in
the freezer for a quick winter lunch or dinner.
Even if you got some non-broccoli fans at your
place, you'll be surprised!

Ingredients

750g broccoli florets
1 litre veggie stock
1/2 cup ground almonds
Sea salt and ground black pepper

Method

Pour the stock and the broccoli florets into a
saucepan, bring to the boil and simmer for
5 – 7 minutes or until just tender. Add the
ground almonds and stir through. Using a
hand blender or food processor, blend until
smooth. Divide into serving bowls and enjoy!

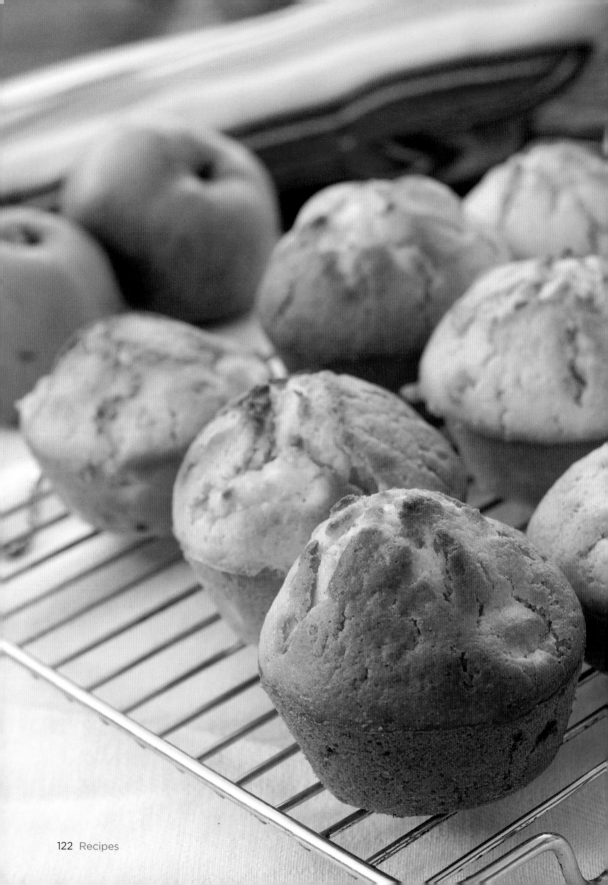

Desserts

Apple Cinnamon Muffins

Muffins are such a comfort food. Enjoy these delicious yet highly nutritious treats!

Ingredients
3 tbsp milk
2 eggs
1/2 cup olive oil
2 tbsp golden syrup
1 cup grated apple
1/4 cup chopped walnuts
1/2 cup almond meal
1 1/4 cups self-raising flour
1/2 tsp ground cinnamon
Butter for greasing

Method
Preheat oven to 180 degrees celcius. Grease two 12 hole muffin tins with butter.

Place milk, eggs, olive oil, golden syrup, grated apple, walnuts and almond meal in a large bowl and stir to combine. Sift in the flour and cinnamon and stir gently until just combined. Spoon the mixture evenly into the prepared muffin tins.

Bake for 25 - 30 minutes or until golden and cooked through. Allow to stand for about 5 minutes, then turn out onto a wire rack to cool.

Apple, Fig and Pecan Slice

Ingredients
Zest of 1 orange
125ml (1/2 cup) orange juice
150g (2/3 cup) raw sugar
150g (1/2 cup) honey
100g (1/2 cup) dried figs, chopped
60g (1/3 cup) raisins
1 apple grated
150g (1 cup) plain flour
150g (1 cup) self-raising flour
1 tsp baking powder
1/2 tsp ground cinnamon
1 tsp mixed spice
2 eggs, lightly beaten
60 ml (1/4 cup) extra virgin olive oil
90g (3/4 cup) pecans, roughly chopped
Cream cheese icing (optional)

Method
Preheat oven to 180° C

Combine orange zest, juice, sugar, honey, figs and raisins in a saucepan. Bring to the boil over a medium heat, then remove and allow to cool. Add the grated apple. Sift the flours, baking powder and spice together and add to mixture. Add eggs, oil and pecans and mix well until combined. Spoon into a lined 22cm cake tin or equivalent slice tin. Bake for 45 minutes. Check with a skewer. If the skewer comes out clean, the slice is cooked, if it doesn't, cook for a further 5 - 10 minutes and check again. Allow to cool in tin for 15 minutes, then remove and cool on a cooling rack.

If desired, beat a carton of light cream cheese with a tablespoon of caster sugar and spread over the slice.

Serves 6 - 8

Banana and Hazelnut Porridge

Ingredients
2 cups whole organic rolled oats
1 litre rice milk (or skim milk)
100g hazelnut meal
1 vanilla bean, halved
2 ripe bananas, mashed

To Serve
1/2 cup rice milk (or skim milk)
Sliced Banana (optional)
Brown sugar or maple syrup (optional)

Method
Place oats, milk and 1 cup water in a saucepan.
Cook, stirring over medium heat for 10 minutes
or until oats are soft and creamy.

Add hazelnut meal, vanilla bean and banana
and cook for a further 5 minutes or until
heated through. Remove vanilla bean.

Serve in bowls with milk, topped with banana,
brown sugar or maple syrup if desired

Serves 4

Honey and Apricot Pots

Healthy, nutritious and delicious, this easy dish
is a family fave!

Ingredients
250g dried apricots
200ml freshly squeezed orange juice
2 tsp honey and a little extra for topping!
170g thick natural yoghurt
1 tbsp almonds, lightly crushed

Method
Place fry pan over medium heat, dry fry the
lightly crushed almonds for 2 – 3 minutes or
until golden. Set aside. Place the apricots,
orange juice and honey in a small saucepan.
Simmer for about 8 – 10 minutes or until
apricots are soft and plump, remove from
heat and set aside to cool. Once cooled, place
the fruit evenly in 4 small serving pots, then
top with the yoghurt and lastly sprinkle with
the toasted almonds and drizzle with honey.
Enjoy!

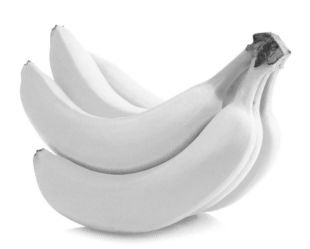

Blueberry Ricotta Pancakes

Yes you can have your pancakes and eat them too! Naughty and nice all in one!

Ingredients

250g ricotta cheese
3/4 cup skim milk
2 tablespoons apple puree
1 cup wholemeal plain flour
1 tsp baking powder
4 eggs
Light olive oil
400g blueberries
Natural yogurt to serve

Method

Place the ricotta, milk and apple puree into a large bowl and mix to combine. Add the flour and the baking powder and stir until just combined. In a separate bowl, whisk the eggs until light and fluffy. Slowly fold the eggs through the flour mixture until just combined. Lightly oil a fry pan with olive oil, pour 1/4 cup of the mixture into the pan and cook over medium heat for 3 minutes or until bubbles appear on the surface. Flip the pancake over and cook the other side until golden. Repeat with remaining mixture. Serve with blueberries and yoghurt. Enjoy!

Blueberry Ricotta Pudding

These light fluffy puddings make a great end to any meal!

Ingredients

100g blueberries
250g ricotta
2 teaspoons honey
2 egg whites, lightly beaten

Method

Preheat oven to 180 degrees Celsius. Line 2 small oven proof bowls (1 cup size), with baking paper. Place half the blueberries into each bowl. Mix the ricotta and honey together in a bowl and mix well. Fold in the egg whites. Once combined spoon the mixture over the berries. Place the bowls onto a baking dish with enough boiling water to come halfway up the side of the bowls. Bake for 15 minutes or until set. Remove from oven and invert onto plates to serve.

Smoothies

Coconut Smoothie

Coconut water is the new 'buzz' drink, used by celebs! This yummy smoothie combines the goodness of coconut water with a good dose of calcium, protein and vitamin C.

Ingredients

1 cup pure coconut water
1 cup natural greek yoghurt
1 cup mango chunks (frozen or fresh)
1/4 orange juice
2 cups ice

Method

Place all ingredients into a blender or food processor and blend until smooth. Pour into a tall chilled glass (ice optional). Enjoy!

Forest Fruit Smoothie

Smoothies are a great way snack for sensitive stomachs during pregnancy, as well as being quick, easy and delicious! This one is a favourite, you can play around with the quantity and type of berries depending on your preference.

Ingredients

1/2 strawberries
1/4 cup blackberries
1/4 cup blueberries
3/4 cup natural yoghurt
3/4 cup skim milk
1 tbsp wheatgerm (optional)

Method

Place all ingredients into a blender or food processor and blend until smooth. Pour into a tall chilled glass (ice optional). Enjoy!

Banana Berry Smoothie

Cottage cheese adds a lovely richness to this tasty smoothie.

Ingredients
1 cup blueberries
1 cup blackberries
(or any combination of 2 cups of your favourite berries)
1 medium ripe banana
1/2 cup low fat cottage cheese
1/2 cup chilled water

Method
Place all ingredients into a blender or food processor and blend until smooth. Pour into a tall chilled glass (ice optional). Enjoy!

Berry Banana Smoothie

Bananas are a good source of the all-important pregnancy nutrient choline and the tofu provides some extra protein in this tasty snack!

Ingredients
1 1/4 cups orange juice
1 medium ripe banana
1 cup blueberries, blackberries or raspberries (fresh or frozen)
1/2 cup silken tofu

Method
Place all ingredients into a blender or food processor and blend until smooth. Pour into a tall chilled glass (ice optional). Enjoy!

Morning Sickness Smoothie

This quick, easy, tasty smoothie provides a great nutrient packed start to the morning whilst also helping to relieve nausea and morning sickness. Nice and gentle on sensitive stomachs.

Ingredients
1 cup (250ml) apple of pear juice
3 fresh or tinned peaches, stone removed and chopped
2 tbsp organic natural yoghurt
1 banana, chopped
1 tsp ginger, finely grated

Method
Pop all ingredients into a blender with a handful of ice, whizz and enjoy!

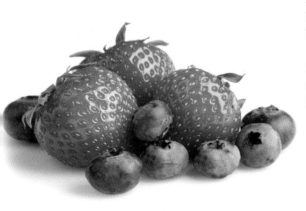

Index

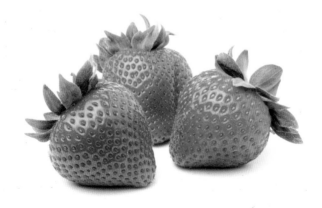